Eat For Life™ By Marsha
Snackalicious
COOKIES, CAKES, CUPCAKES, AND MORE
GLUTEN-FREE & DAIRY-FREE

Marsha Hebert

Copyright © 2020 by Marsha Hebert

Eat For Life By Marsha Snackalicious
was created and published by Marsha Hebert
Printed in Canada

ISBN 978-0-9950959-1-5

Cooking: Healthy & Healing
Cookbooks

All rights reserved. No part of this work covered by the copyrights hereon may be reproduced or used in any form or by an means – graphic, electronic or mechanical – or stored in a retrieval system or transmitted in any form by any means without the prior written permission of the publisher. except for reviewers, who may quote brief passages. Any request for photocopying, recording, taping or storage on information retrieval systems of any part of this work shall be directed in writing to the publisher.

This book is intended as general information only and should not be used to diagnose or treat any health condition. The ideas, procedures, and suggestions in this book are intended to supplement, not replace, the advice of a trained medical professional. The author and publisher disclaim any liability arising directly or indirectly from the use of this book.

Always follow safety and common-sense cooking protocol while using kitchen utensils, operating ovens, and stoves, and handling uncooked food.

This book is available at quantity discounts for bulk purchases. For information, please email eatforlifebymarsha@gmail.com.

THANK YOU

I hope as you read, you will feel inspired by my recipes to help you Eat For Life!

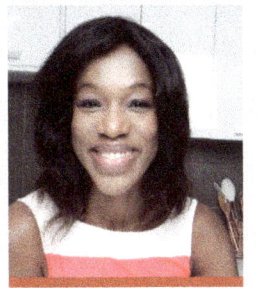

My mission: to develop delicious, nutritious, gluten-free, dairy-free, cornstarch-free, and yeast-free recipes; create meals in minutes that support a healthier, happier you. Find **Eat For Life By Marsha** recipes in my magazines, cookbooks, on website, and social media.

My passion for cooking and baking has its roots in my Jamaican childhood, helping my mom to cook delicious and nutritious meals made from whole foods in her home-based restaurant. When I came to Canada at age 12, cooking with whole foods continued with my Stepmom, who is Portuguese. This included lots of seafood and the opportunity to learn about Portuguese cuisine. I was diagnosed with anemia, suffered with gut issues, acne, depression, anxiety, and increased body fat for many years. I was unaware I had food intolerances with gluten, wheat, dairy, yeast, and cornstarch.

When I became a mother in 1991, my daughter had developed issues due to my lack of proper nutrition. I wanted to be there for my child, and to find healthy ways to improve my daughter's cognitive ability. It was difficult to find budget¬-friendly, nutritious, and convenient ready-made foods, so I returned to cooking the way I did growing up in Jamaica, and with my stepmom - using mostly natural foods. Later, I enrolled in the Canadian School of Natural Nutrition and completed the Fundamentals of Nutrition. I am currently pursuing certification to become a Certified Nutritional Consultant.

I am fully committed to creating recipes that improve our health and increase nutrient-rich foods in our daily meals.

I believe that **what we eat should make us healthier and happier.**

From my kitchen to yours, let's Eat For life!

MARSHA HEBERT
Author & Publisher

Eat For Life By Marsha

Snackalicious
COOKIES, CAKES, CUPCAKES, AND MORE
GLUTEN-FREE & DAIRY-FREE

CONTENTS

Nutrients Essential For Life, **4**
Ingredients Essential Foods, **5**
Cooking Equivalent Measurement, **74**

COOKIES

1. Almond Pumpkin Seed Cookies, **7** GRAIN-FREE | KETO | PALEO | VEGETARIAN
2. Almond Chocolate Raspberry Filling Cookies, **9** GRAIN-FREE | PALEO | VEGAN | VEGETARIAN
3. Sesame Tahini Red Beet Cookies, **11** GRAIN-FREE | KETO | PALEO | VEGETARIAN
4. Almond Coconut Cranberry Chocolate Chip Cookie, **13** VEGAN | VEGETARIAN
5. Carrot Raisin-Pecan Cookie, **15** VEGETARIAN
6. Pecan Oat Cookies, **17** VEGAN | VEGETARIAN
7. Carrot Chocolate Chip Cookies, **19** GRAIN-FREE | PALEO | VEGAN | VEGETARIAN
8. Blueberry Almond Cookies with Cashew Blueberry Filling, **21** GRAIN-FREE | PALEO | VEGAN | VEGETARIAN
9. Almond Cherry Coconut Cookies, **23** GRAIN-FREE | PALEO | VEGETARIAN

CAKES

1. Fig Cranberry Almond Cake, **25** GRAIN-FREE | VEGETARIAN
2. Chocolate Zucchini Cake, **27** GRAIN-FREE | PALEO | VEGETARIAN
3. Almond Pumpkin Spice Cake, **29** GRAIN-FREE | PALEO | VEGETARIAN
4. Whoopie Cakes With Cranberry Cashew Filling, **31** GRAIN-FREE | VEGAN | VEGETARIAN
5. Apple and Peanut Cake Squares, **33** GRAIN-FREE | PALEO | VEGETARIAN
6. Carrot Walnut and Raisin Cake, **35** VEGETARIAN
7. Blueberry Almond Coffee Cake, **37** GRAIN-FREE | PALEO | VEGETARIAN

CUPCAKES

1. Almond Pecan Mini Cupcakes, **39** GRAIN-FREE | VEGETARIAN
2. Pumpkin Seed, Coconut, & Kiwi Cupcakes, **41** GRAIN-FREE | PALEO | VEGETARIAN
3. Double Chocolate and Black Bean Cupcakes, **43** VEGETARIAN
4. Raspberry Cupcake with Avocado Cranberry Frosting, **45** GRAIN-FREE | PALEO | VEGETARIAN
5. Peanut and Banana Mini Cupcakes, **47** VEGETARIAN

AND MORE

1. Caramel Pecan Cranberry Coconut Popcorn, **49** VEGAN | VEGETARIAN
2. Brown Rice Crisp and Trail Mix Treats, **51** VEGAN | VEGETARIAN
3. Fig Oat Mini Donuts, **53** VEGAN | VEGETARIAN
4. Fig Oat Scones, **55** VEGAN | VEGETARIAN
5. Pumpkin Seed Cranberry Mix Oat Squares, **57** VEGAN | VEGETARIAN
6. Apple Betty, **59** VEGAN | VEGETARIAN
7. Potato Oat and Cheese Muffins, **61** VEGETARIAN
8. Prune Plum and Oat Muffins, **63** VEGETARIAN
9. Vegan Chocolate Chickpea and Peach Muffins, **65** VEGETARIAN
10. Duchess Potatoes with Kale, **67** GRAIN-FREE | VEGETARIAN
11. Corn Puffs with Kale and Bell Pepper, **69** GRAIN-FREE | VEGETARIAN
12. Asparagus Hummus, **71** GRAIN-FREE | VEGAN | VEGETARIAN

you got this

you got this

you got this

Image source: Canva

NUTRIENTS
ESSENTIAL FOR LIFE

Are you getting enough vitamins, minerals and acids that work together for a healthy body and mind?

FAT-SOLUBLE VITAMINS

A (retinol/beta carotene)	D (calciferol)	E (tocopherol)	K
Regulates the immune system and helps protect against bacteria and viruses. Helps night vision.	Helps maintain levels of calcium and phosphorus in the blood.	In alpha-tocopherol form helps protect against several cancers and may help protect against hay fever and asthma.	Helps blood clot, Also, helps the healthy functioning of the kidney, aids bone growth and repair.

WATER-SOLUBLE VITAMINS

C (ascorbic acid)	B1 (thiamine)	B2 (riboflavin)	B3 (niacin)
Vital for healthy immune functioning. Protects against heart disease, and aids tissue growth and wound healing.	Improves circulation, digestion and brain function.	Helps maintain healthy skin, nails and hair. Essential for production of red blood cells.	Regulates blood sugar levels, lowers cholesterol and improves circulation.

B6 (pyridoxine)	B12 (cobalamin)	Folic Acid (B9)	Biotin (B7)
Keeps the immune and nervous systems healthy.	Helps maintain healthy nerve cells and red blood cells.	In alpha-tocopherol form helps protect against several cancers and may help protect against hay fever and asthma	Essential for the utilization of fats and amino acids, and helps keep skin nails and hair healthy.

MINERALS

Calcium (Ca)	Magnesium (Mg)	Phosphorus (P)	Potassium (K)
A vital role in growth of strong bones, gums and teeth. Also, keeps your heat working healthy.	Maintains muscle and nerve functioning, and keep bones strong. Helps the body process fats and protein.	An essential mineral needed for every cell in the body. Mostly used in bones.	Helps the body store blood sugar in the form of glycogen, which is the principal source of energy required by all muscles in the body.

Sulfur (S)	Chromium (Cr)	Copper (Cu)	Iron (Fe)
Key role in the manufacture of amino acids and in the conversion of carbohydrates to a form that the body can use.	Helps insulin bind to its receptors on the membrane of body cells, then allow for the sugar glucose to move into the cells for energy production.	The production of pigment in skin, hair, and eyes; the development of healthy bones, teeth and heart. Processing of iron and formation of red blood cells	A component of hemoglobin (the oxygen-carrying protein in red blood cells), it plays a key role in transporting oxygen around the body.

Selenium (Se)	Zinc (Zn)	Sodium (Na)	Iodine (I)
Vital for the normal functioning of the immune system and the thyroid gland.	Essential for the breakdown of carbohydrates, fats, and proteins. Also, necessary to maintain normal levels of the male hormone (testosterone).	Controls the amount of water in the body, maintains the normal pH of blood, transmits nerve signals and helps muscle contractions.	Used for making thyroid hormones, which are required for normal body metabolism and growth.

ACIDS

Coenzyme Q10 Non-Essential Fatty Acids	Omega-3 (fish oils) Essential Fatty Acids	Omega-6 (vegetable oils) Essential Fatty Acids
May improve blood pressure and vascular function..	Provide calories to give your body energy and have many functions in your heart, blood vessels, lungs, immune system.	Used for reducing the risk of heart disease, lowering "bad" (LDL) cholesterol levels, raising "good" (HDL) cholesterol levels.

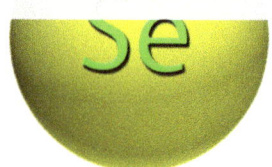

Image source: Canva

INGREDIENTS
ESSENTIAL FOODS

Essential ingredients mean eating a nutritious diet primarily acquiring all the vitamins, minerals, amino acids, fatty acids, and phytonutrients that the body needs to function optimally for a healthy body and mind. Eating specific foods that contain good levels of many nutrients includes fruits, vegetables, wlhole grains, lelgumes, nuts, and seeds.

NUTS AND SEEDS

NUTRIENTS
calcium, fibre, flavonoids, folate, iron, magnesium, manganese, monounsaturated, fats, omega-3 fatty acids, potassium, protein, selenium, vitamin E, Zinc

HELPFUL HEALING
diabetes, cardiovascular disease, high cholesterol, cancer, low energy, constipation, anemia, weight gain

FRUITS AND VEGETABLES

NUTRIENTS
beta-carotene, fibre, flavonoids, folate, iron, magnesium, potassium, vitamin A, C

HELPFUL HEALING
diabetes, cardiovascular disease, high cholesteroJ, cancer, low energy, constipation

WHOLESOME GRAINS

NUTRIENTS
B vitamins, complex carbohydrates, fibre, folate, iron, magnesium, vitamin E, zinc

HELPFUL HEALING
diabetes, cardiovascular disease, cancer, digestive health, anemia

Image source: Canva

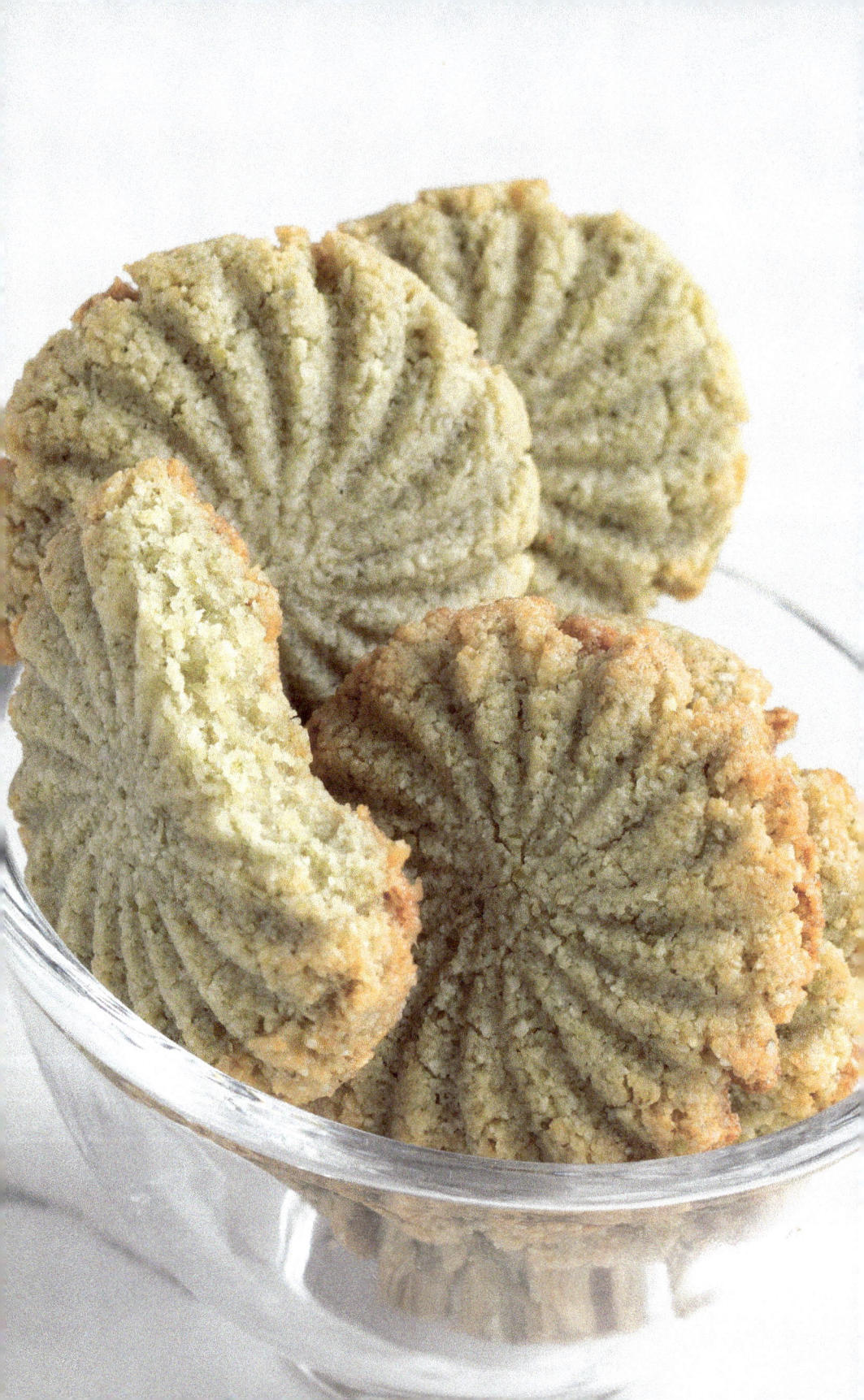

Almond Pumpkin Seed Cookies

TIME: 12 - 15 MINUTES | MAKES: 14 COOKIES

Ingredients

- 1-3/4 cups (155 grams) blanched almond flour
- 3/4 cup (105 grams) pumpkin seeds, grounded
- 1/2 cup (90 grams) erythritol sweetener
- 1/2 teaspoon (2 grams) baking powder
- 1/4 teaspoon (1 gram) salt
- 1 large egg
- 1/3 cup (65 grams) coconut oil, melted but not hot
- 1/2 teaspoon (2 grams) almond extract

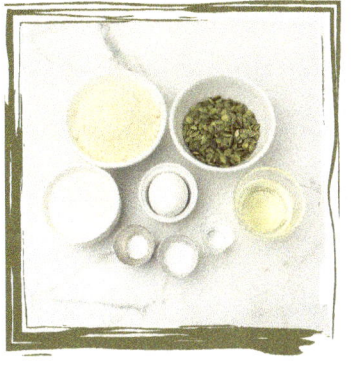

Instructions

1. Preheat the oven at 325F (160C). Line cookie baking pan with parchment paper or leave ungreased.
2. To ground pumpkin seeds, in a food processor, add the pumpkins seeds, process until very finely chopped. Set aside.
3. In a medium bowl, whisk together the almond meal, erythritol sweetener, baking powder, and salt. Add the grounded pumpkin seeds. Set aside
4. In a large mixing bowl, add the egg, coconut oil, almond extract. Blend to combine with electric mixer. Stir in the almond flour mixture until dough combines.
5. Place Shape dough into 1-inch balls, place 2 inches apart on cookie pan. Slightly flatten. Bake 12 - 15 minutes, until the edges are firm and lightly golden. Remove from the oven and let stand for 5 minutes onto cookie pan. Transfer to a wire rack and let cool. Serve and enjoy!

GRAIN-FREE | KETO | PALEO | VEGETARIAN

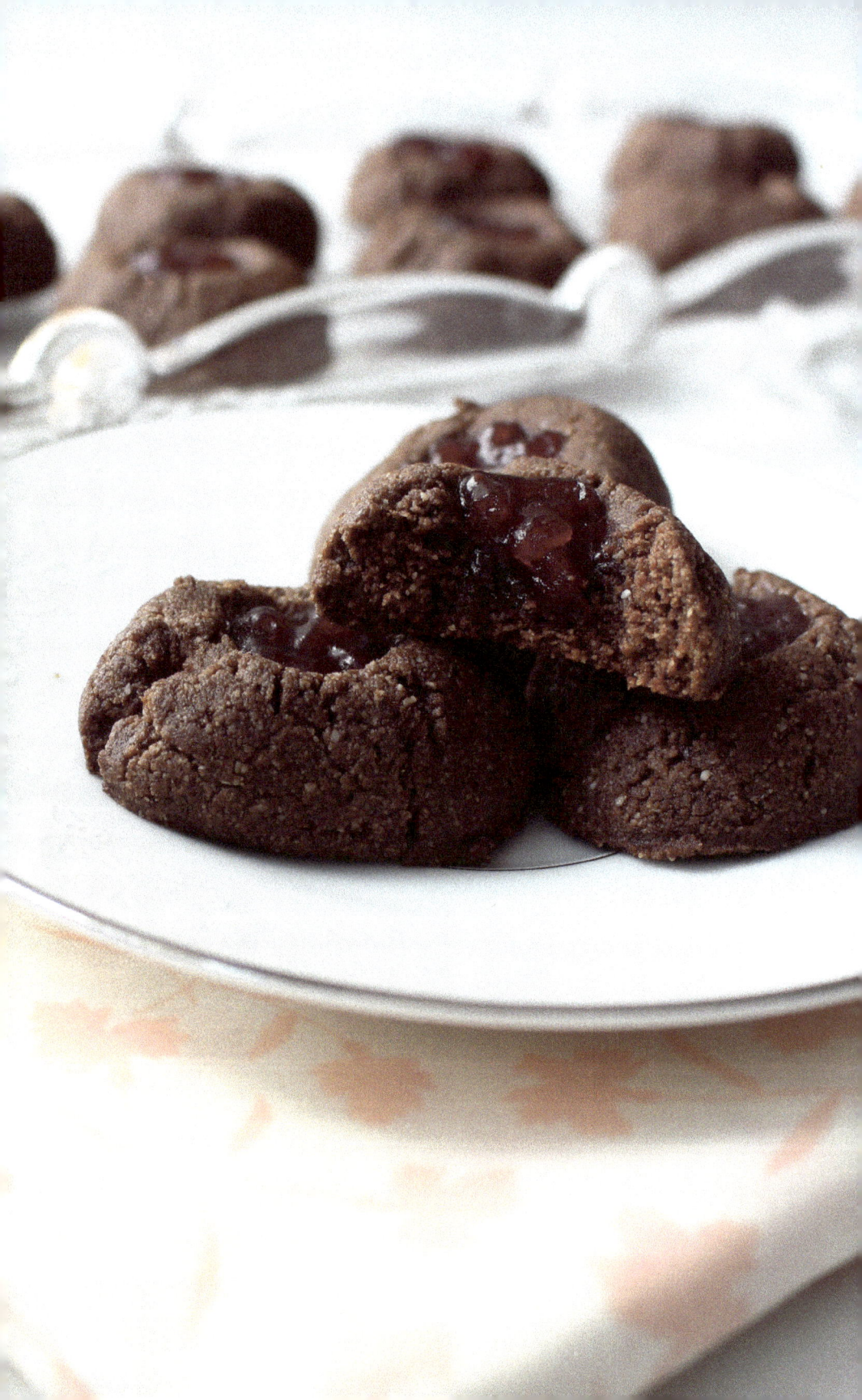

Almond Chocolate Raspberry Filling Cookies

TIME: 12 - 15 MINUTES | MAKES: 16 COOKIES

Ingredients

- 1/3 cup (65 grams) vegan butter, room temperature
- 1/4 cup (50 grams) brown sugar
- 1/4 cup (25 grams) cacao powder
- 1-1/2 cups (165 grams) almond meal
- 1/4 cup (60 grams) raspberry preserves (1/2 teaspoon per cookie)

Instructions

1. Make sure oven rack is in middle of oven and then preheat oven to 325F (160C). Grease or line cookie baking pan with parchment paper.
2. In a medium bowl, cream butter and 1/3 cup brown sugar with an electric mixer until creamy. Sift in cacao powder blend with mixer. Add almond meal until completely blended.
3. Use a small cookie scoop or a 1-tablespoon measure to add balls of cookies onto prepared
4. baking sheet. Press the middle of cookie with your thumb, add 1/2 teaspoon of raspberry preserves to each cookie.
5. Bake 10 - 15 minutes. Remove from oven and let cool on cookie sheet for 5 minutes. Transfer to wire rack to cool completely. Serve and enjoy!

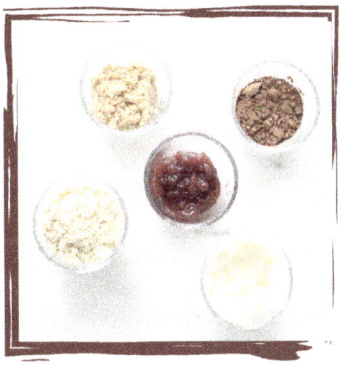

GRAIN-FREE | PALEO | VEGAN

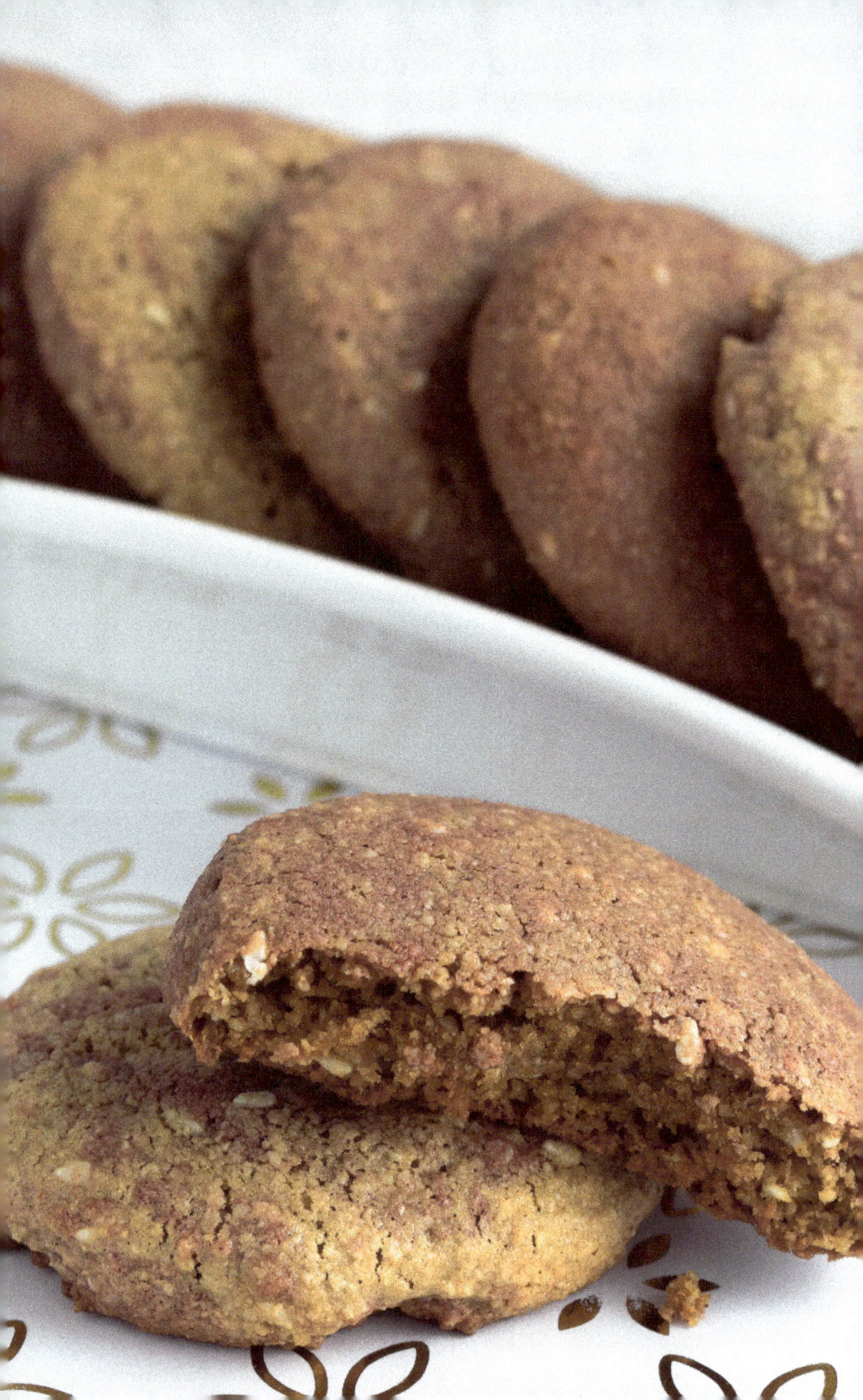

Sesame Tahini Red Beet Cookies

TIME: 12 - 15 MINUTES | MAKES: 18 COOKIES

Ingredients

- 1-1/2 cups (150 grams) blanched almond flour
- 2 tablespoons (20 grams) sesame seeds
- 1/2 teaspoon (2 grams) baking soda
- 1/4 teaspoon salt (1 gram)
- 2 large eggs
- 1/2 cup (120 grams) tahini
- 2/3 cups (100 grams) coconut sugar
- 1 teaspoon (4 grams) vanilla extract
- 1 tablespoon (12 grams) red beet powder

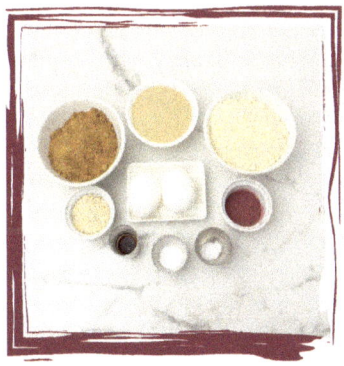

Instructions

1. Preheat the oven at 325F (160C). Grease or line cookie baking sheet with parchment paper.
2. In a medium bowl, whisk together the almond meal, sesame seeds, baking soda, and salt. Set aside
3. In a large mixing bowl, add the eggs, tahini, coconut sugar, and vanilla. Blend to combine with electric mixer. Stir in the almond flour mixture until dough combines. Blend in beet powder or follow directions in next step for beet swirl.
4. For the beet swirl: In a medium bowl, reserve half (240 grams) of the dough. Add the beet powder to the mixing bowl and blend until combined. Add the reserved dough and lightly fold in to create the swirl.
5. Using a cookie scoop or tablespoon, place dough 2 inches apart on cookie baking sheet. Slightly flatten. Bake 12 - 15 minutes, until the edges are firm and lightly golden. Remove from the oven and let stand for 5 minutes onto cookie pan. Transfer to a wire rack and let cool. Serve and enjoy!

GRAIN-FREE | KETO | PALEO | VEGETARIAN

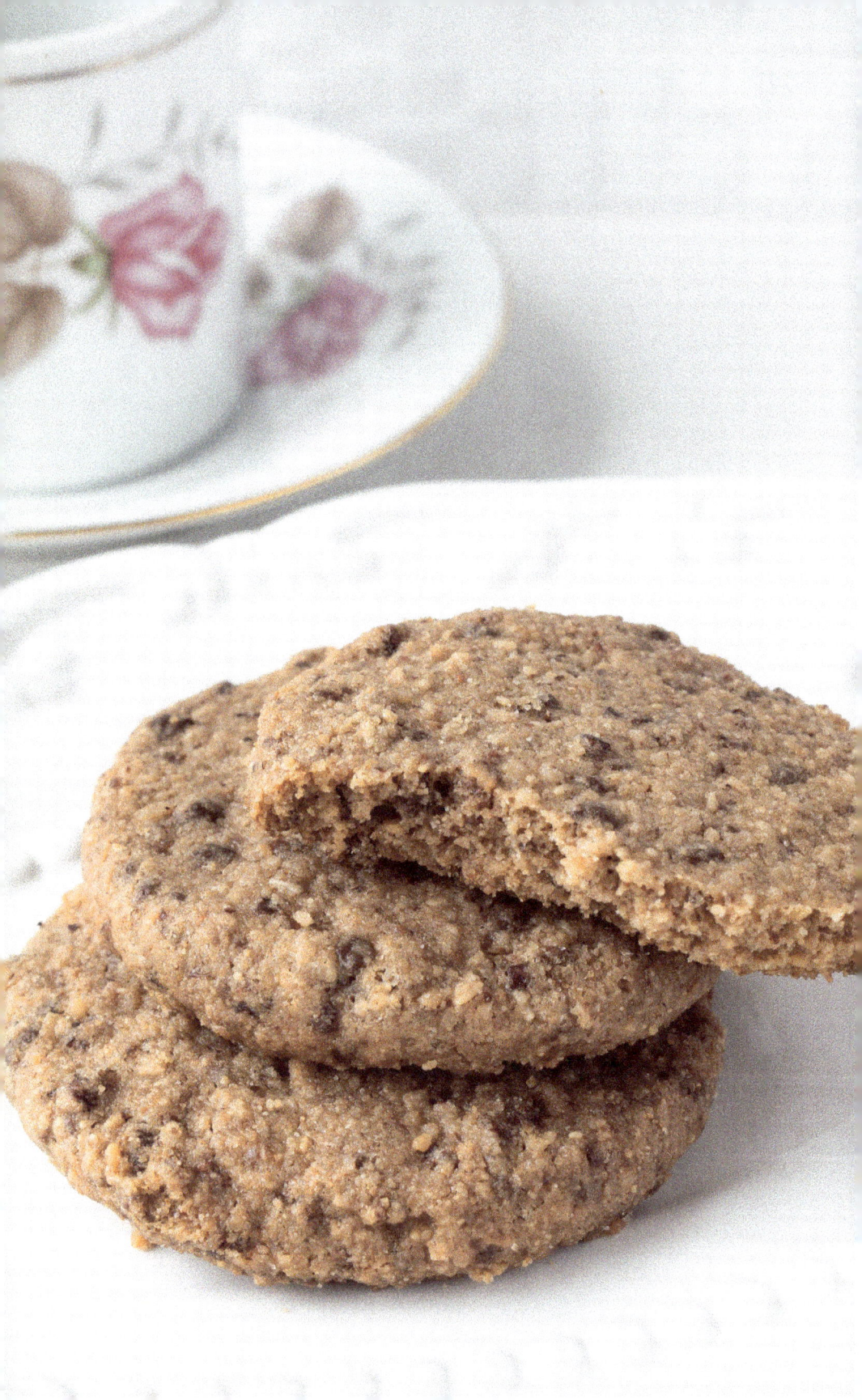

Almond Coconut Cranberry Chocolate Chip Cookie

TIME: 12 MINUTES | MAKES: 16 COOKIES

Ingredients

- 1/4 cup (35 grams) shredded coconut
- 1/3 cup (40 grams) dried cranberries
- 1/2 cup (80 grams) vegan chocolate chips
- 1 cup (130 grams) brown rice flour
- 1/2 teaspoon (2 grams) baking soda
- 1/4 teaspoon (1 gram) salt
- 1/2 cup (120 grams) almond butter, raw or roasted
- 1/3 cup (45 grams) brown sugar
- 1/2 cup (50 grams) coconut oil
- 1/2 teaspoon (2 grams) almond extract

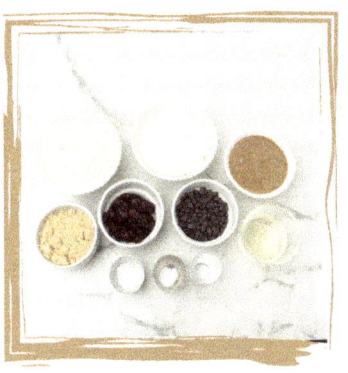

Instructions

1. Preheat the oven at 325F (160C). Line cookie baking pan with parchment paper or leave ungreased.
2. In a food processor, combine the coconut, cranberries, and chocolate chips. Process until very finely chopped. Set aside.
3. In a medium bowl, whisk together the brown rice flour, baking soda, and salt. Set aside
4. In a large mixing bowl, add the almond butter, coconut oil, and almond extract. Beat with an electric mixer until combined, scraping sides of bowl occasionally. Stir in the flour mixture and then the coconut mixture. Mix until combined.
5. Place Shape dough into 1-inch balls, place 2 inches apart on cookie pan. Slightly flatten. Bake 12 - 15 minutes, until the edges are firm and lightly golden. Remove from the oven and let stand for 5 minutes on cookie pan. Transfer to a wire rack and let cool. Serve and enjoy!

VEGAN | VEGETARIAN

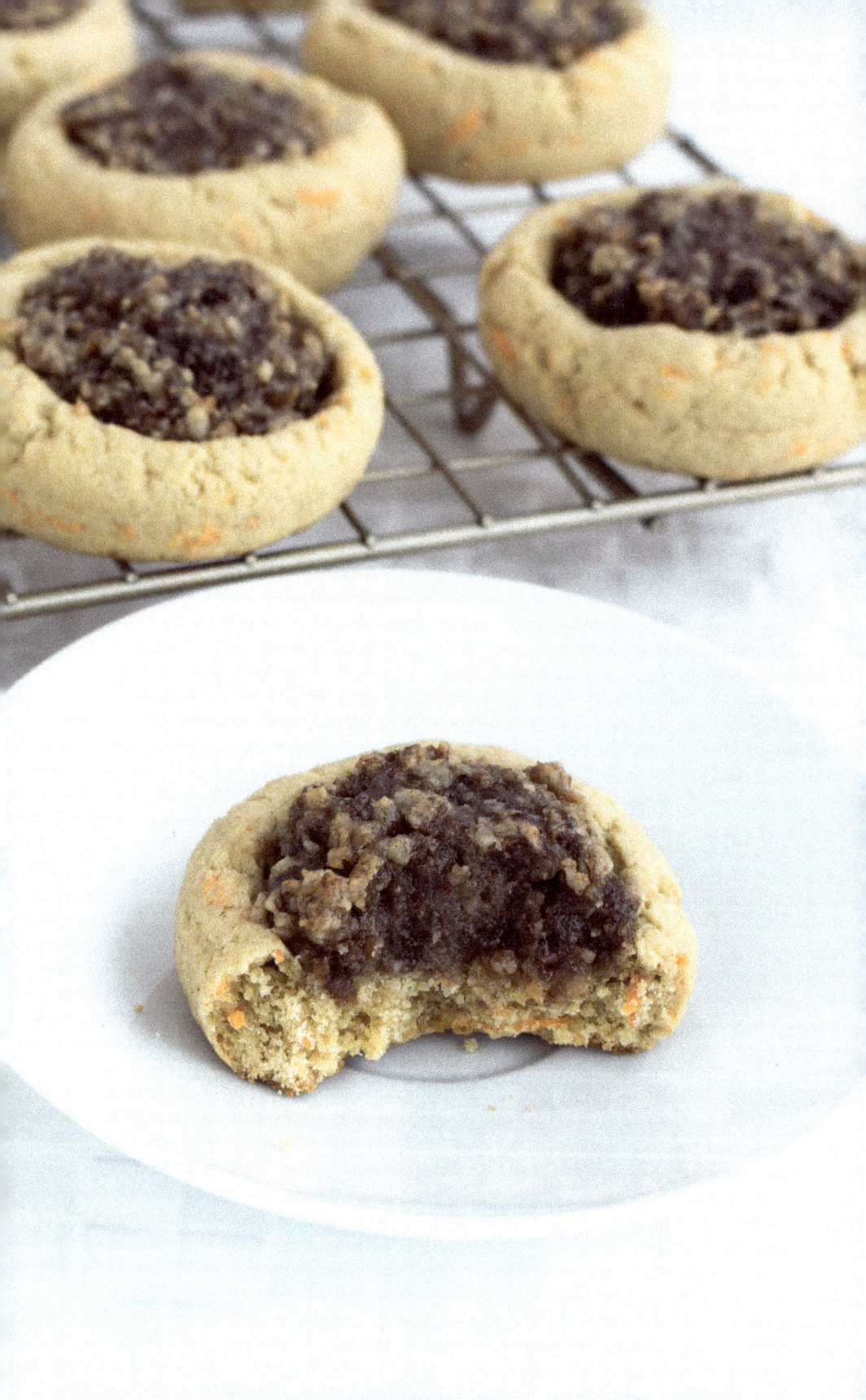

Carrot Raisin-Pecan Cookie

TIME: 12 MINUTES | MAKES: 18 COOKIES

Ingredients

Cookie Filling
- 1/3 cup (55 grams) raisins
- 1/2 cup (50 grams) pecans
- 2 tablespoons (40 grams) maple syrup

Cookie Dough
- 1/2 cup (95 grams) vegan butter, softened
- 1/2 cup (90 grams) granulated sugar
- 1/4 teaspoon (1 gram) baking powder
- 1/4 teaspoon (1 gram) salt
- 1 large egg
- 2-1/3 cups (250 grams) oat flour
- 1/2 cup (40 grams) finely shredded carrots

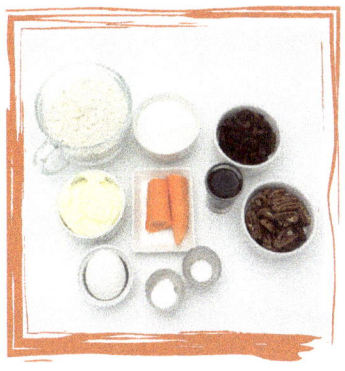

Instructions

To Make The Filling
1. In a food processor, combine the raisins, pecans, and maple syrup. Process until very finely chopped. Pour into a small bowl and set aside.

To Make The Cookie
1. Preheat the oven at 375F (190C). Grease or line cookie baking pan with parchment paper.
2. In a large mixing bowl, beat the butter with an electric mixer on medium to high speed for 30 seconds. Add sugar, baking powder, and salt. Beat until combined, scraping sides of bowl occasionally. Beat in egg until combined. Beat in as much of the oat flour as you can. Stir in remaining flour, add carrots, and mix until combined.
3. Shape dough into 1-inch balls, place 2 inches apart on cookie pan. Make an indentation in the centre of each ball, add 1 teaspoon of the raisin-pecan filling to each cookie.
4. Bake 10 – 12 minutes, until the edges are firm and lightly golden. Remove from the oven and let stand for 1 minute on cookie pan. Transfer to a wire rack and let cool. Serve and enjoy!

VEGETARIAN

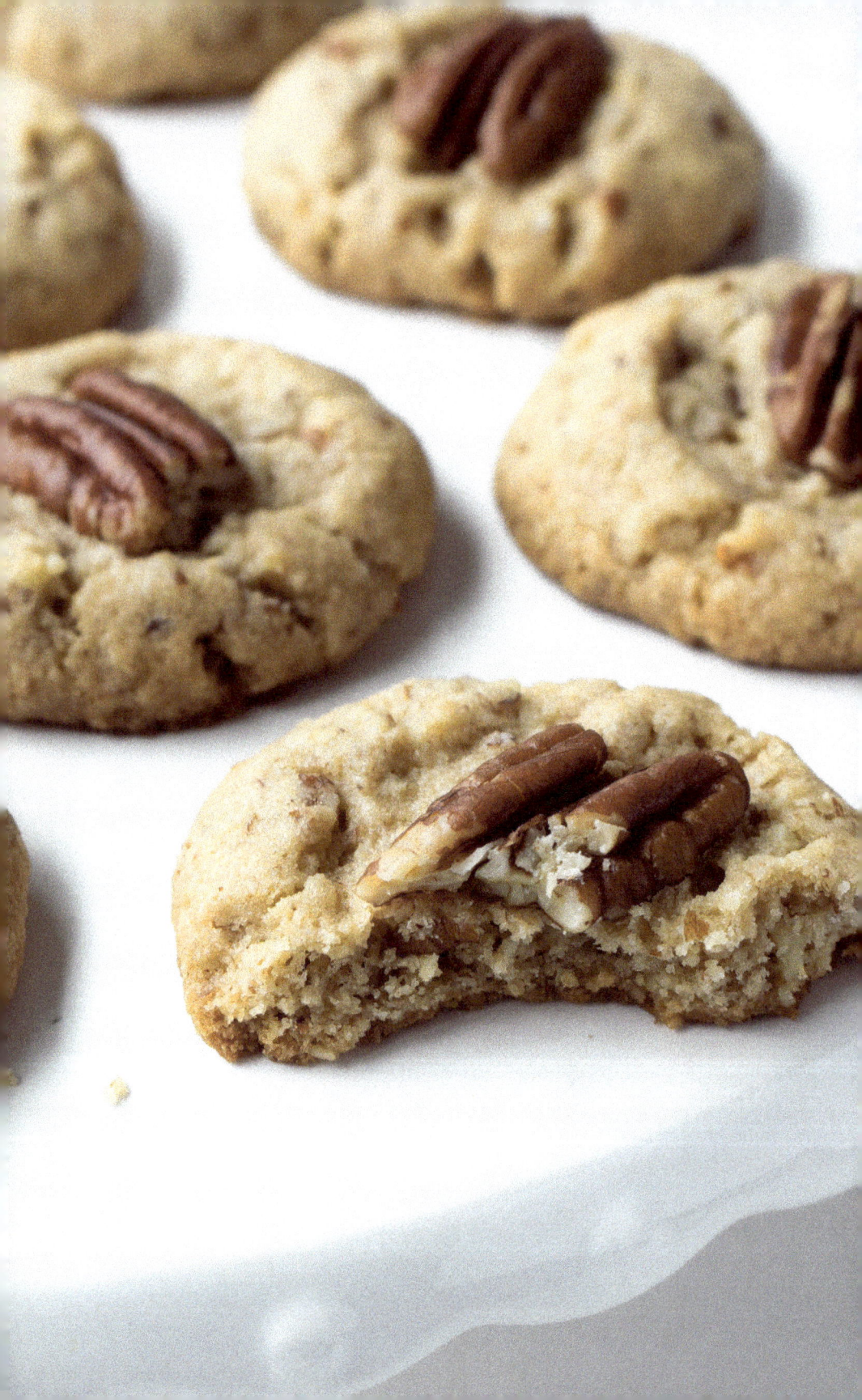

Pecan Oat Cookies

TIME: 14 MINUTES | MAKES: 16 COOKIES

Ingredients

- 1/2 cup (115 grams) vegan butter unsalted, room temperature
- 1/3 cup (70 grams) brown sugar
- 1 teaspoon (4 grams) vanilla extract
- 1/8 teaspoon salt
- 1 1/3 cup (145 grams) oat flour
- 3/4 cup (80 grams) pecans, finely chopped

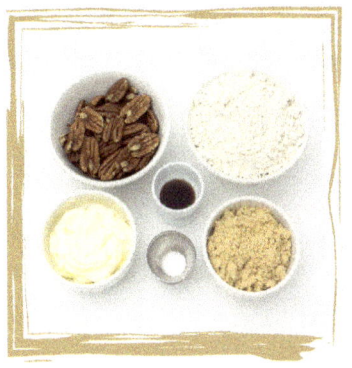

Instructions

1. Preheat oven at 350F (180C). Lightly grease cookie baking pan or line with parchment paper.
2. In a large bowl, add the butter, beat with an electric mixer on high for about 1 minute. Add sugar and beat until light, about 1 minute. Beat in vanilla, salt, and oat flour. just until dough comes together. Fold in pecans.
3. Using a cookie scoop or tablespoon measure, place dough on baking pan about 3 inches apart. Roll into balls, add pecan halves, pressing lightly to flatten mounds of dough.
4. Bake for 14 minutes, rotating baking pan halfway through for evenly baking. Remove from oven, cool in pan for 5 minutes, then transfer to wire rack for further cooling. Serve and enjoy!

VEGAN | VEGETARIAN

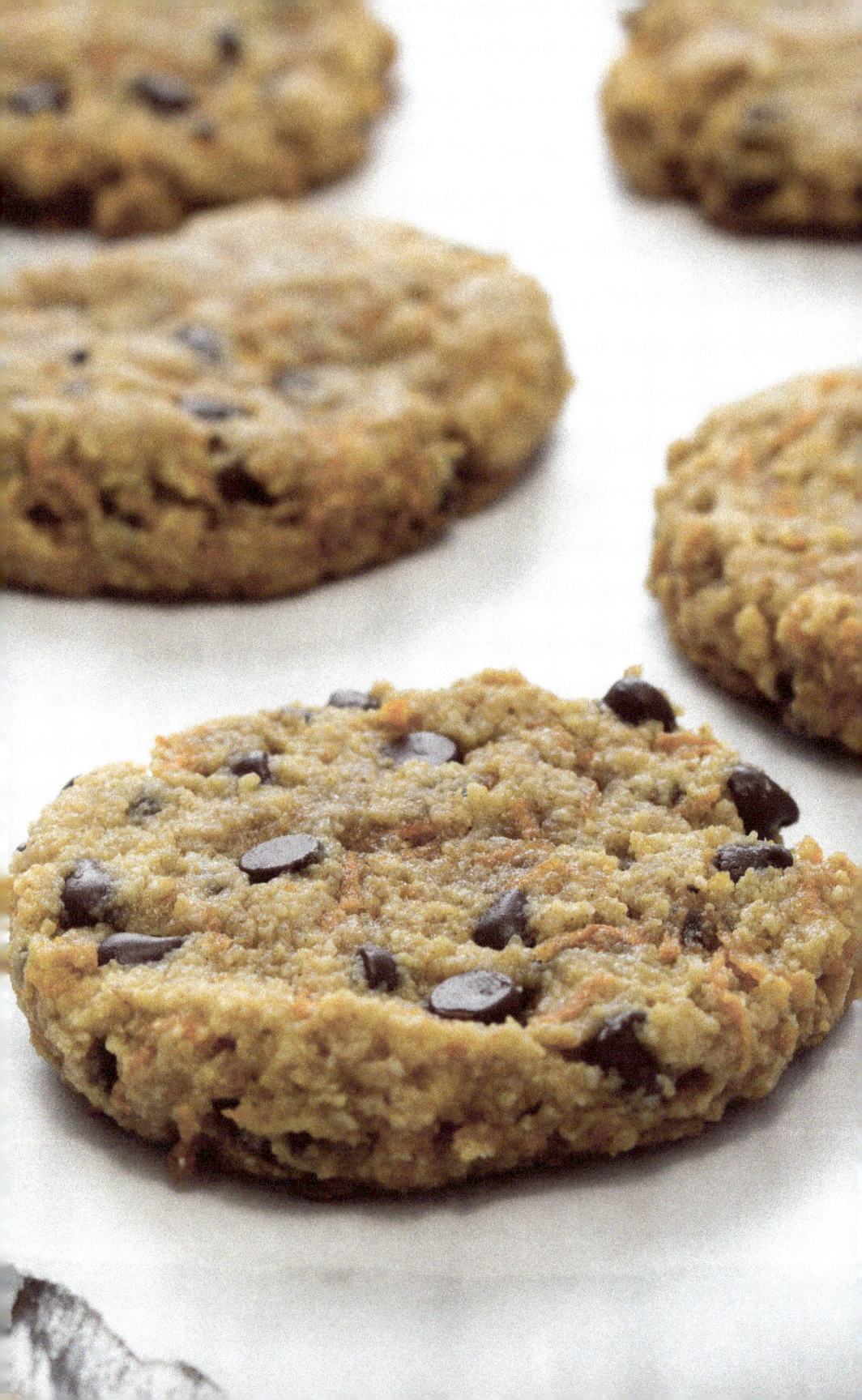

Carrot Chocolate Chip Cookies

TIME: 15 MINUTES | MAKES: 16 COOKIES

Ingredients

- 1/2 cup (125 grams) smooth natural peanut butter
- 1/4 cup (70 grams) maple syrup
- 1 teaspoon (3 grams) vanilla extract
- 1 cup (110 grams) almond meal
- 1/8 teaspoon salt
- 1/3 cup (65 grams) vegan mini chocolate chips
- 3/4 cup (80 grams) finely grated carrots

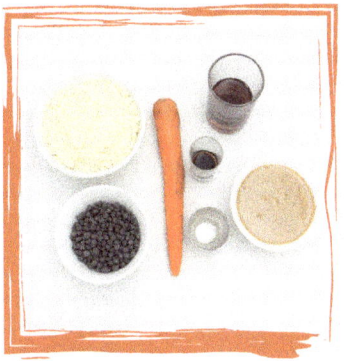

Instructions

1. Preheat oven to 350F (180C). Grease cookie pan or line with parchment paper.
2. In a large bowl, add the peanut butter, maple syrup and vanilla; stir with spatula until completely combined. Add the almond meal and salt, mix to combined. Then gently stir in chocolate chips and carrots
3. Use cookie scoop or tablespoon measure and place mixture onto prepared baking, slightly flatten. Bake for 15 minutes or until golden brown. Let cool on baking pan for 2 minutes then transfer to wire rack to cool completely. Serve and enjoy

GRAIN-FREE | PALEO | VEGAN | VEGETARIAN

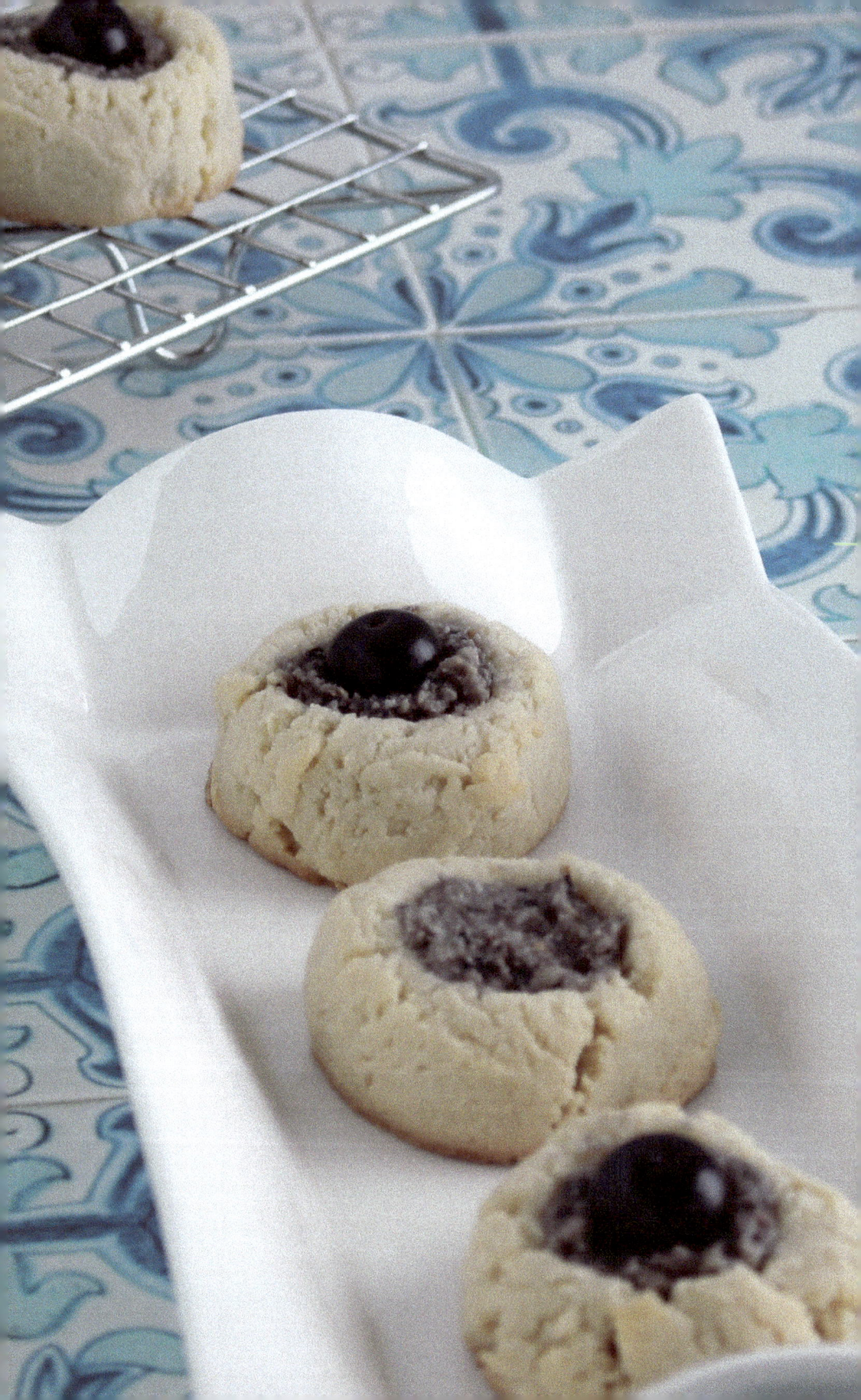

Blueberry Almond Cookies with Cashew Blueberry Filling

TIME: 20 MINUTES | MAKES: 24 COOKIES

Ingredients

Cookie Filling
- 1/3 cup (50 grams) fresh blueberries
- 3/4 cup (110 grams) raw cashews
- 2 tablespoon (40 grams) maple syrup

Cookie Dough
- 1/3 cup (70 grams) vegan butter, melted and cooled
- 1/4 cup (80 grams) maple syrup
- 1/2 teaspoon (1 gram) almond extract
- 1/8 teaspoon salt
- 2-1/2 cups (280 grams) almond meal

Instructions

To Make The Filling
1. In a food processor, combine the blueberries, cashews, and maple syrup. Process until very finely chopped. Pour into a small bowl and set aside.

To Make The Cookie
1. Preheat the oven at 3250F (160C). Grease or line cookie baking pan with parchment paper.
2. In a large mixing bowl, beat the butter with an electric mixer on medium to high speed for 30 seconds. Add maple syrup, almond extract, and salt. Beat until combined, scraping sides of bowl occasionally. Beat almond meal until combined.
3. Shape dough into 1-inch balls, place 2 inches apart on cookie pan. Make an indentation in the centre of each ball, add 1 teaspoon of the blueberry-cashew filling to each cookie.
4. Bake 15 - 20 minutes, until the edges are firm and lightly golden. Remove from the oven and let stand for 1 minute on cookie pan. Transfer to a wire rack and let cool. Serve and enjoy!

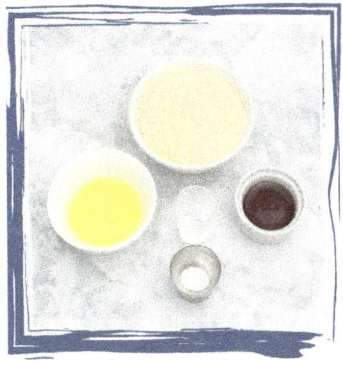

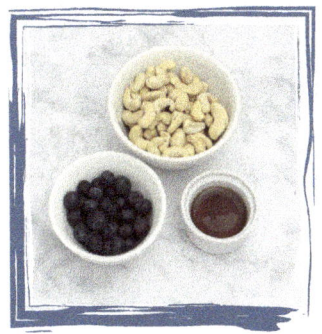

GRAIN-FREE | PALEO | VEGAN | VEGETARIAN

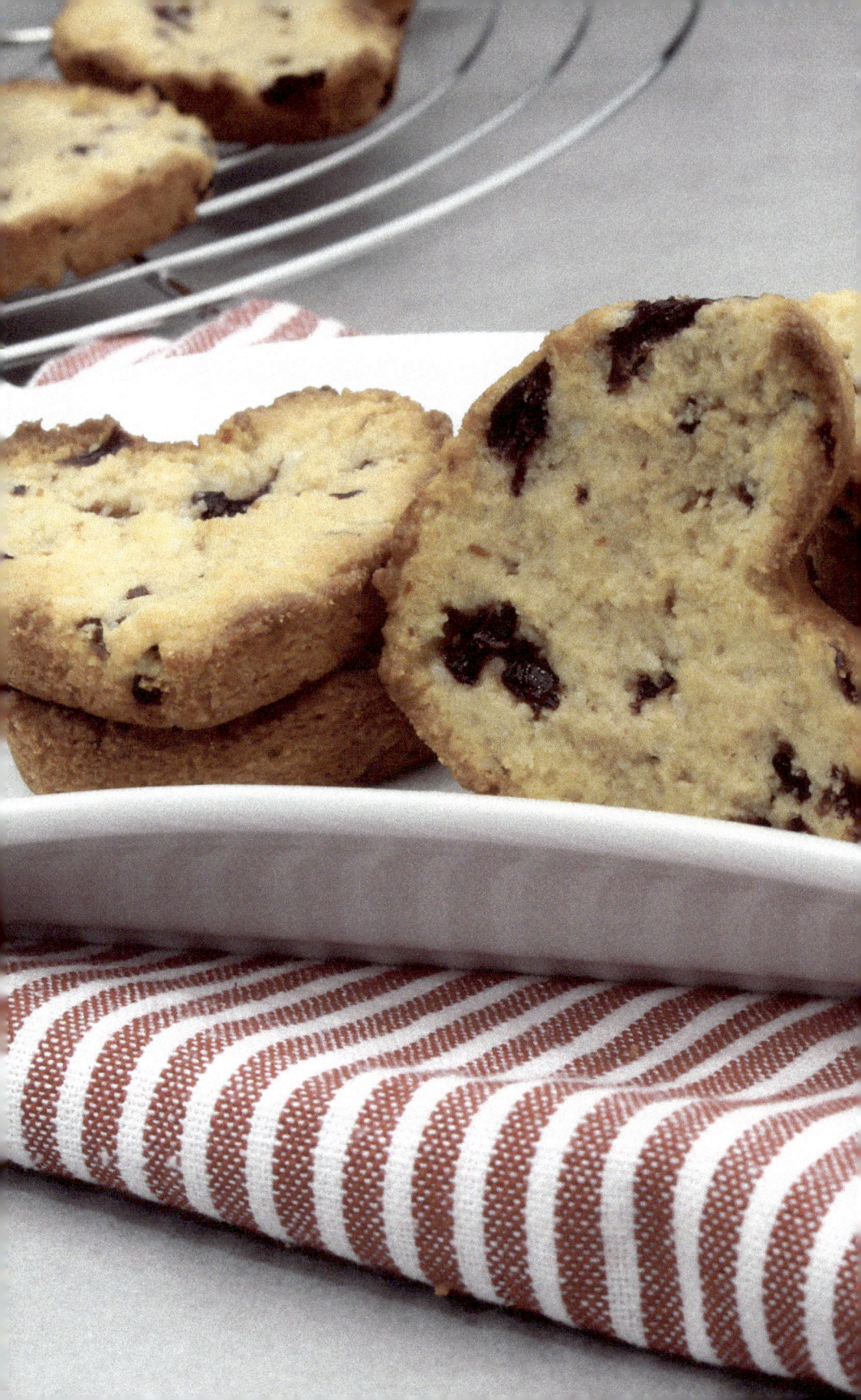

Almond Cherry Coconut Cookies

TIME: 12 MINUTES | MAKES: 24 COOKIES

Ingredients

- 1 -1/2 cups (145 grams) almond meal
- 1 cup (95 grams) shredded coconut
- 1/8 teaspoon salt
- 1/4 cup (55 grams) butter
- 1/3 cup (55 grams) brown sugar
- 1 large egg
- 1 teaspoon (2 grams) vanilla extract
- 1/2 cup (85 grams) finely chopped cherries, fresh or frozen (thaw, drain excess liquid)

Instructions

1. Make sure oven rack is in middle of oven and then preheat oven to 350F (180C). Grease or line cookie baking pan with parchment paper.
2. In a medium bowl, combine the almond meal, coconut and salt. Set aside.
3. In a large bowl, cream butter and sugar. Beat in the egg. Beat in the vanilla extract. Gradually stir in the dry ingredients. Fold in the cherries.
4. Using a cookie scoop or tablespoon, place the dough 1-inch apart on prepared baking pan. Bake for 10 – 12 minutes, until lightly golden brown. Remove from oven, let cool in pan for 2 minutes then transfer to wire to cool completely. Serve and enjoy!

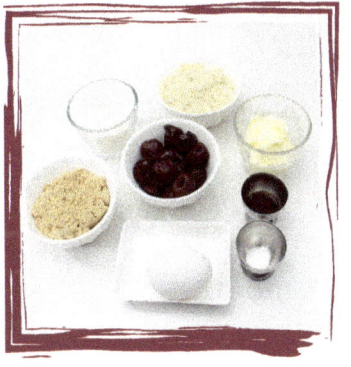

GRAIN-FREE | PALEO | VEGETARIAN

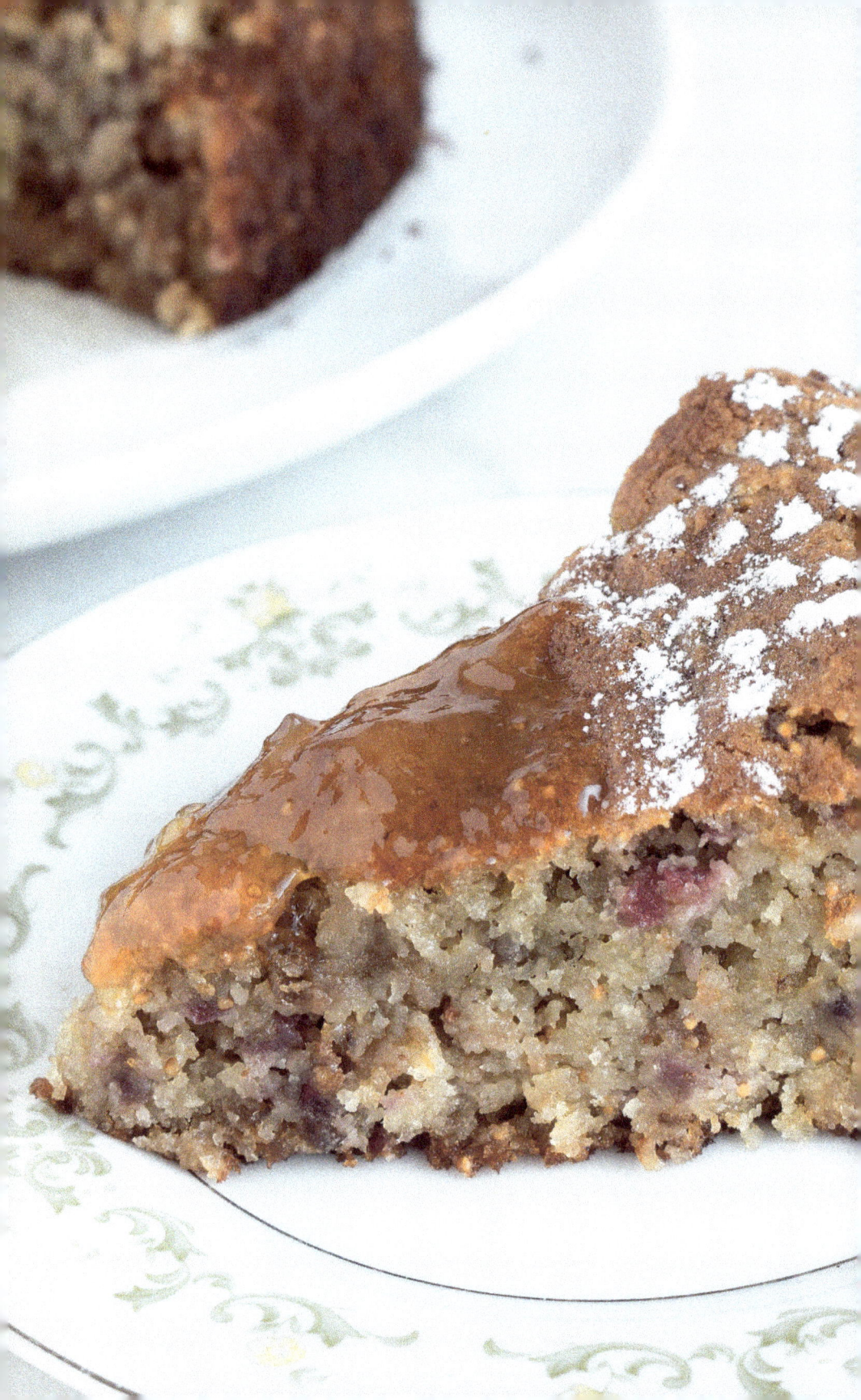

Fig Cranberry Almond Cake

TIME: 45 MINUTES | MAKES: 8-INCH CAKE

Ingredients

- 1 cup (170 grams) dried figs
- 1/2 cup (106 grams) boiling water
- 1 cup (100 grams) cranberries, fresh or frozen thawed
- 2-1/2 cups (280 grams) blanched almond flour
- 1 teaspoon (4 grams) baking powder
- 1/2 teaspoon (2 grams) baking soda
- 1/4 teaspoon (1 gram) salt
- 2/3 cup (145 grams) granulated sugar
- 1/3 cup (90 grams) dairy-free plain yogurt
- 1/4 cup (55 grams) canola oil
- 1/2 teaspoon (1 gram) almond extract
- 3 large eggs

Instructions

1. In a small bowl, combine figs and boiling water; set aside for 30 minutes; drain water. In a food processor, add the figs and cranberries and finely chopped. Set aside.
2. Preheat the oven at 325F (160C). Grease an 8-inch spring-form cake pan. Line the bottom of pan with parchment paper.
3. In a medium bowl, whisk together the almond flour, baking powder, baking soda, and salt. Set aside.
4. In a large mixing bowl, add the sugar, yogurt, oil, and almond extract. Blend to combine with electric mixer. Add the eggs one at a time and beat well after each addition. Beat in the almond flour mixture in two additions until dough combines. Stir in the fig mixture.
5. Pour batter into prepared baking pan and smooth the top. Bake for 40 – 45 minutes, until the cake is golden brown, and the top is firm to the touch. A tester inserted in the centre should come out clean. Remove from oven and let cool in the pan for 10 – 20 minutes . Serve and enjoy!

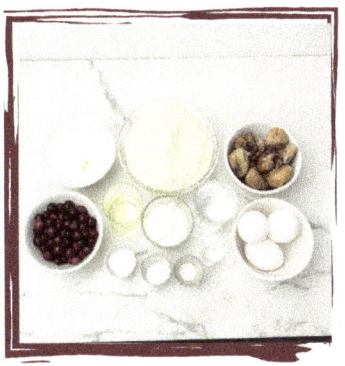

VEGETARIAN | GRAIN-FREE

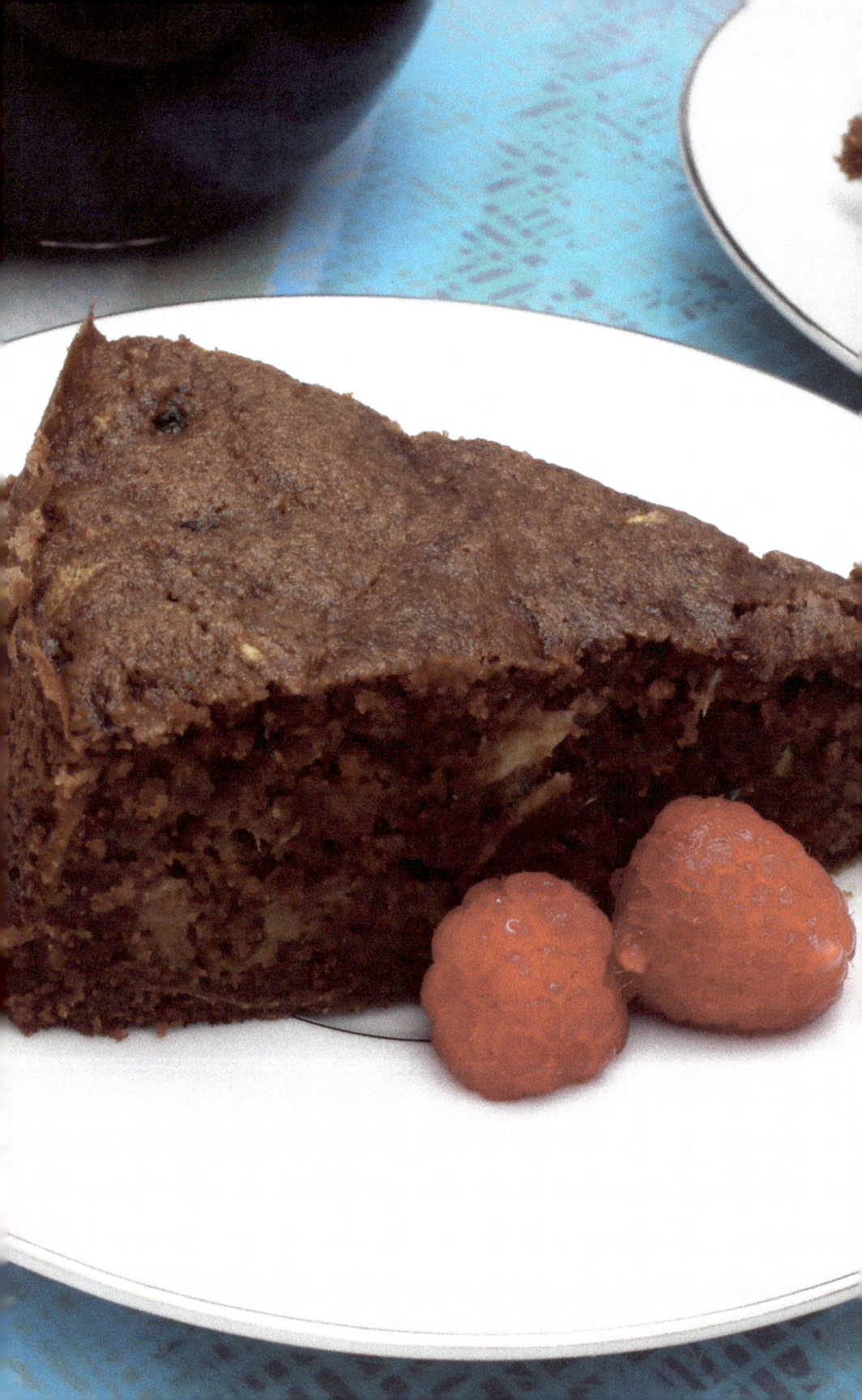

Chocolate Zucchini Cake

TIME: 30 MINUTES | MAKES: 8-INCH CAKE

Ingredients

- 2 cups (210 grams) almond meal
- 1/3 (35 grams) cup cacao powder
- 2 teaspoon (10 grams) baking powder
- 1/8 teaspoon salt
- 3/4 cup (100 grams) brown sugar
- 1/3 cup (65 grams) vegan butter, room temperature
- 3 large eggs, room temperature
- 1 1/2 cups (140 grams) shredded zucchini

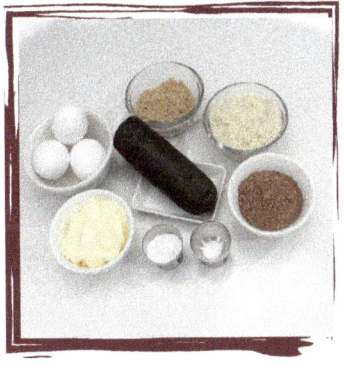

Instructions

1. In a small bowl, combine figs and boiling water; set aside for 30 minutes; drain water. In a food processor, add the figs and cranberries and finely chopped. Set aside.
2. Preheat the oven at 325F (160C). Grease an 8-inch spring-form cake pan. Line the bottom of pan with parchment paper.
3. In a medium bowl, whisk together the almond flour, baking powder, baking soda, and salt. Set aside.
4. In a large mixing bowl, add the sugar, yogurt, oil, and almond extract. Blend to combine with electric mixer. Add the eggs one at a time and beat well after each addition. Beat in the almond flour mixture in two additions until dough combines. Stir in the fig mixture.
5. Pour batter into prepared baking pan and smooth the top. Bake for 40 – 45 minutes, until the cake is golden brown, and the top is firm to the touch. A tester inserted in the centre should come out clean. Remove from oven and let cool in the pan for 10 – 20 minutes . Serve and enjoy!

GRAIN-FREE | PALEO | VEGETARIAN

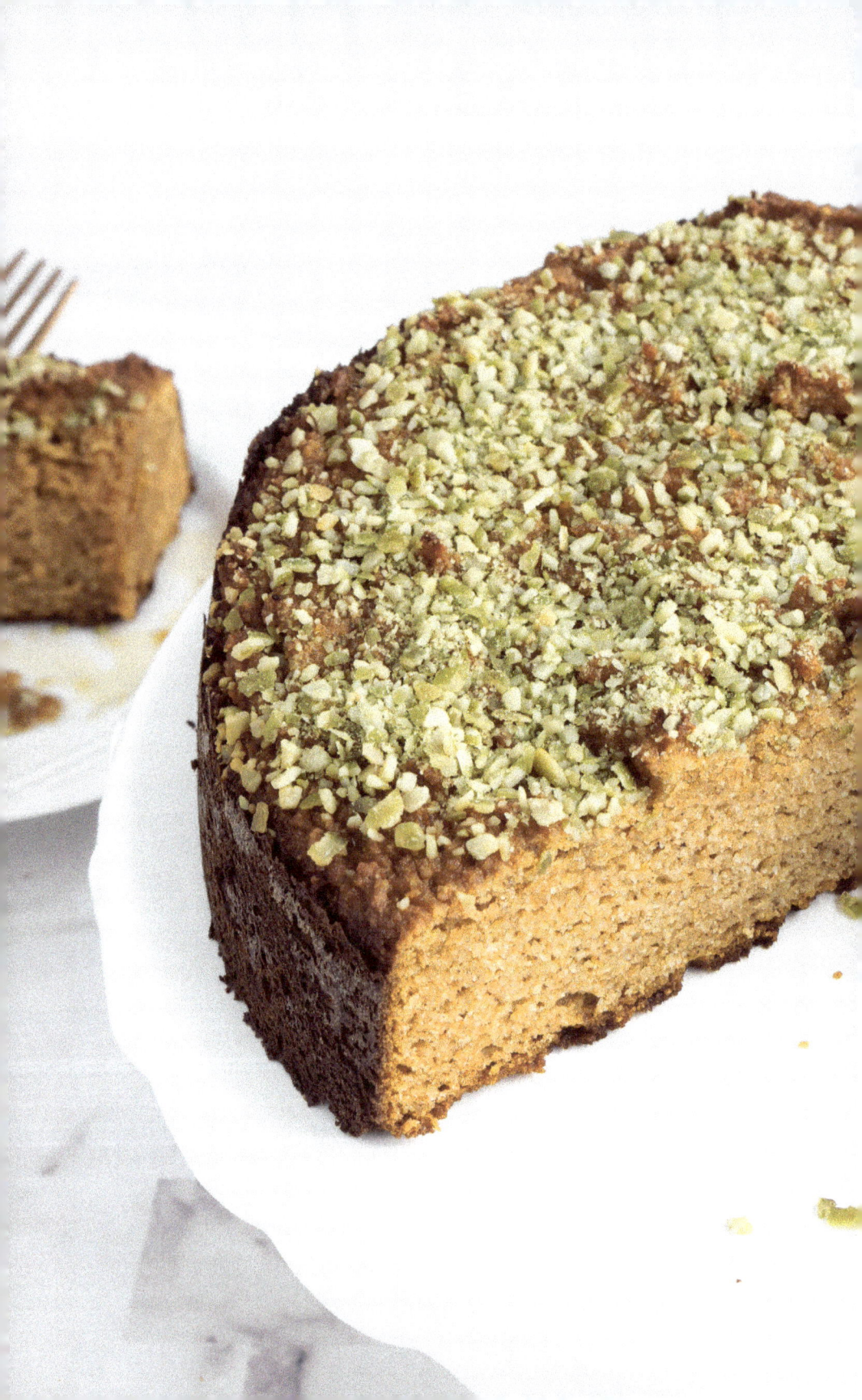

Almond Pumpkin Spice Cake

TIME: 35 MINUTES | MAKES: 8-INCH CAKE

Ingredients

- 2 cups (210 grams) blanched almond flour
- 3 tablespoons (24 grams) coconut flour
- 1-1/2 teaspoons (3 grams) pumpkin pie spice
- 1 teaspoon (5 grams) baking soda
- 14 teaspoon (1 gram) salt
- 3/4 cup (190 grams) pumpkin puree
- 1/2 cup (120 grams) honey
- 2 tablespoons (26 grams) coconut oil, melted
- 4 large eggs
- 2 teaspoons (8 grams) vanilla extract
- 1 teaspoon (3 grams) apple cider vinegar
- Topping Optional
- 1/4 cup finely chopped pumpkin seeds

Instructions

1. Preheat oven at 350F (180C). Grease a 8-inch cake pan and line bottom with parchment paper, slightly grease.
2. In a large bowl, whisk together the almond meal, coconut flour, pumpkin pie spice, baking soda, and salt. Set aside.
3. In a large mixing bowl, add the pumpkin puree, honey, and coconut oil. Using an electric mixer or stand mixer, blend together until smooth and creamy.
4. Add the eggs and vanilla to the pumpkin mixture and blend until well combined.
5. Add the almond flour mixture to the pumpkin mixture and blend until batter is thick and smooth, making sure to scrape down the bowl as needed. Mix in the apple cider.
6. Pour batter into the prepared baking pan using a rubber spatula to scrape all the batter from the bowl. Bake for 35 – 40 minutes, until golden brown and a toothpick inserted int centre comes out clean. let cool in pan for 10 minutes before serving.

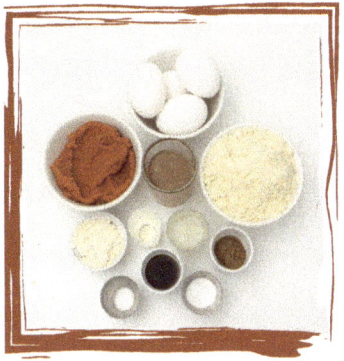

GRAIN-FREE | PALEO | VEGETARIAN

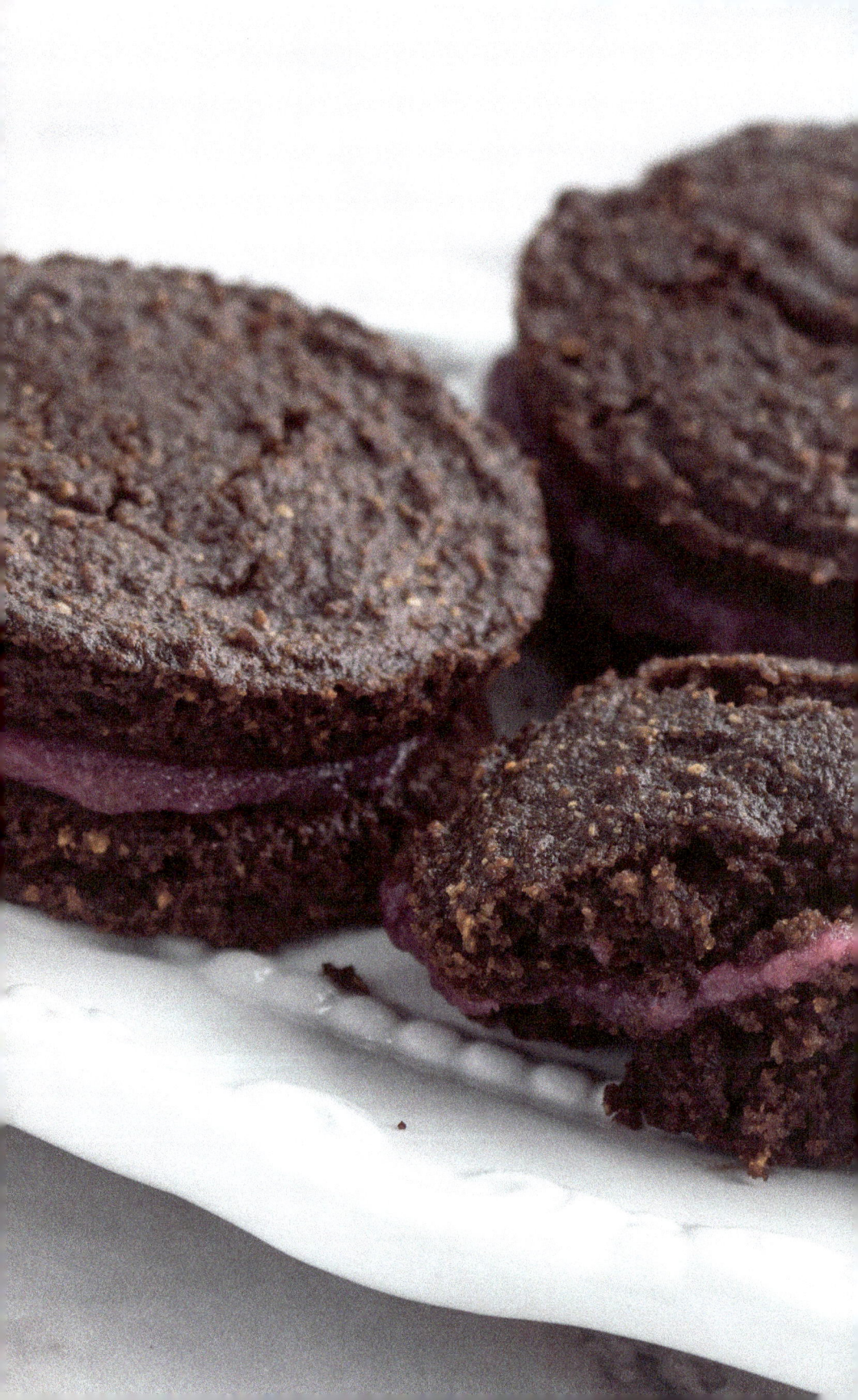

Whoopie Cakes With Cranberry Cashew Filling

TIME: 15 MINUTES | MAKES: 12 CAKES

Ingredients

- 1-1/4 cup (135 grams) almond meal
- 1/3 cup (30 grams) cocoa powder
- 1/4 cup (30 grams) ground flax seeds
- 1/2 cup (75 grams) brown sugar
- 2 teaspoons (10 grams) baking powder
- 1/4 teaspoon (1 grams) salt
- 1/2 cup (45 grams) unsweetened applesauce
- 1/4 cup (45 grams) coconut oil or canola oil
- 1 teaspoon (4 grams) vanilla extract

Filling

- 2 cups (200 grams) fresh or frozen cranberries (thaw if frozen)
- 2 cups (300 grams) raw cashews
- 2/3 cup (130 grams) melted coconut oil
- 1/2 cup (140 grams) maple syrup

Instructions

1. Preheat oven at 325F (160C). Grease a 12-pan whoopie pan.
2. In a large bowl, combine the almond meal, cocoa powder, flax seed, baking powder, and salt. Set a side.
3. In a medium bowl, whisk together the brown sugar, applesauce, oil, and vanilla. Add to centre of almond meal mixture and stir until combined.
4. Pour the batter into the prepared baking pan using a ice cream scoop or 2 tablespoons. Bake for 15 – 17 minutes, or until risen and just firm to the touch. Cool for 5 minutes, then carefully transfer to a cooling rack and let cool completely.

For the filling

1. Place all ingredients into a food process and puree until smooth.
2. To assemble, spread or pipe the filling onto the underside of the whoopie cake and topping with another. Repeat with remaining cakes. Serve and enjoy!

CAKES

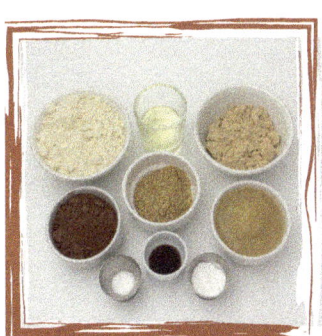

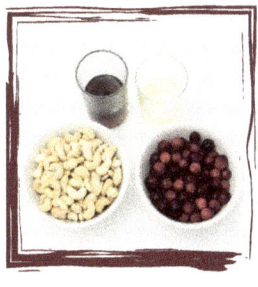

**VEGAN
VEGETARIAN
GRAIN-FREE**

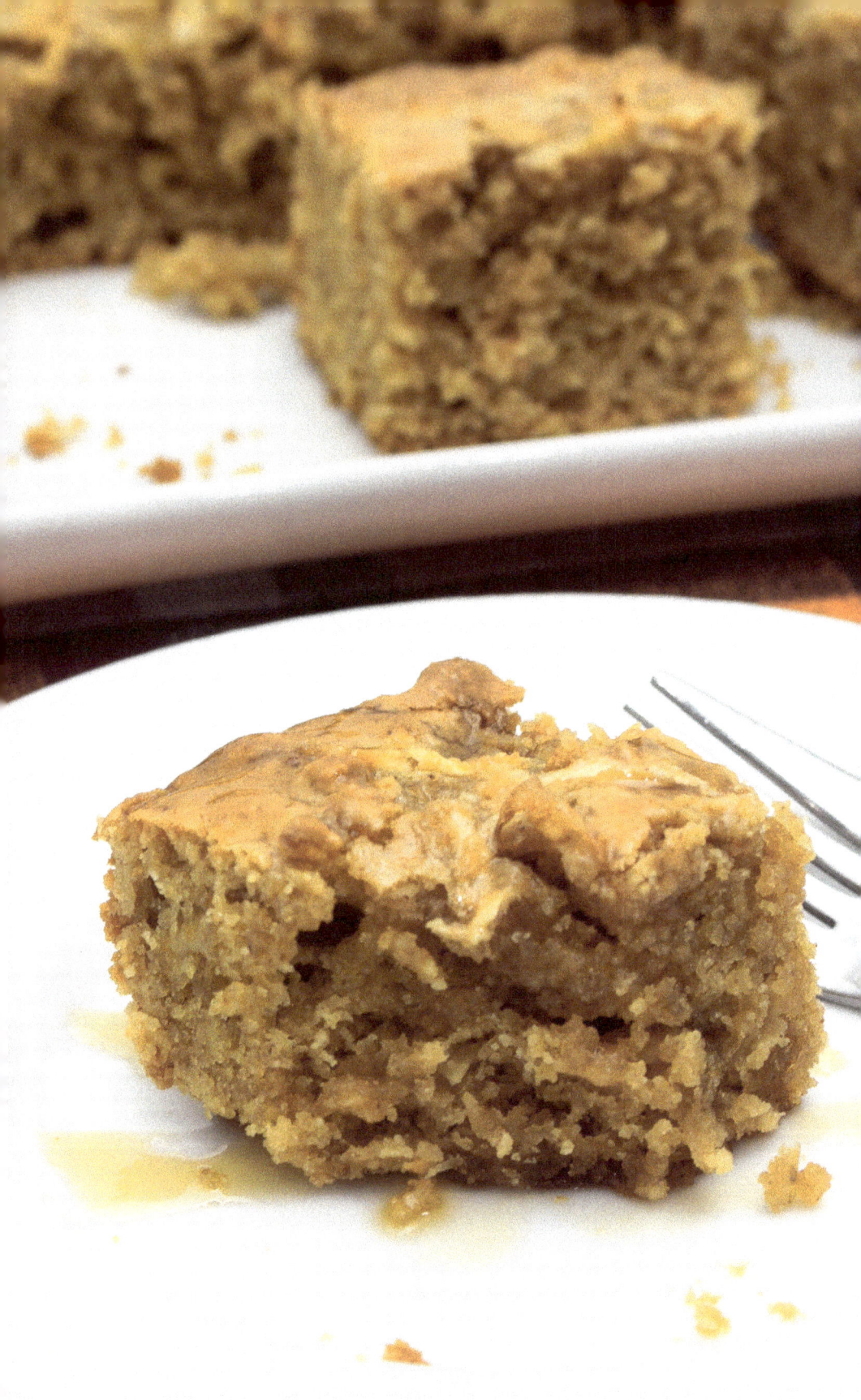

Apple and Peanut Cake Squares

TIME: 35 MINUTES | MAKES: 16 SQUARES (2-INCH X 2-INCH)

Ingredients

- 1-1/2 cups (170 grams) blanched almond flour
- 1/3 cup (25 grams) peanut butter powder
- 2 teaspoons (8 grams) baking powder
- 1/8 teaspoon salt
- 1 (70 grams) apple
- 1/2 cup (120 grams) smooth peanut butter
- 3/4 cup (115 grams) brown sugar
- 3 large eggs, beaten
- 1 teaspoon (3 grams) vanilla extract

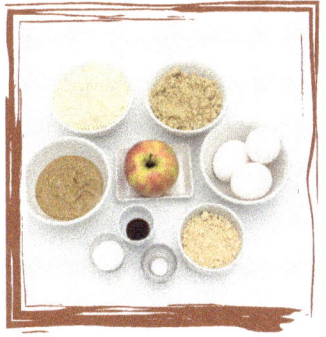

Instructions

1. Preheat the oven at 350F (180C). Grease and line an 8-inch square baking pan.
2. In a medium bowl, mix the almond flour, peanut butter powder, baking powder, and salt. Set aside
3. Peel and grate the apple using the large side of the grater. Set aside with 1/4 cup reserved for topping if desired.
4. In a large mixing bowl, using an electric hand mixer, beat the peanut butter, eggs, and vanilla. Add the almond flour mixture and beat well until the mixture is smooth. Stir in the apples.
5. Pour batter mixture into the prepared baking pan and smooth the surface with spatula. For topping, spread evenly the reserved apples. Bake for 35 – 40 minutes, or until risen, firm, and golden brown. Let cool in the pan for about 10 minutes, then transfer to wire rack to finish cooling. Serve and enjoy!

GRAIN-FREE | PALEO | VEGETARIAN

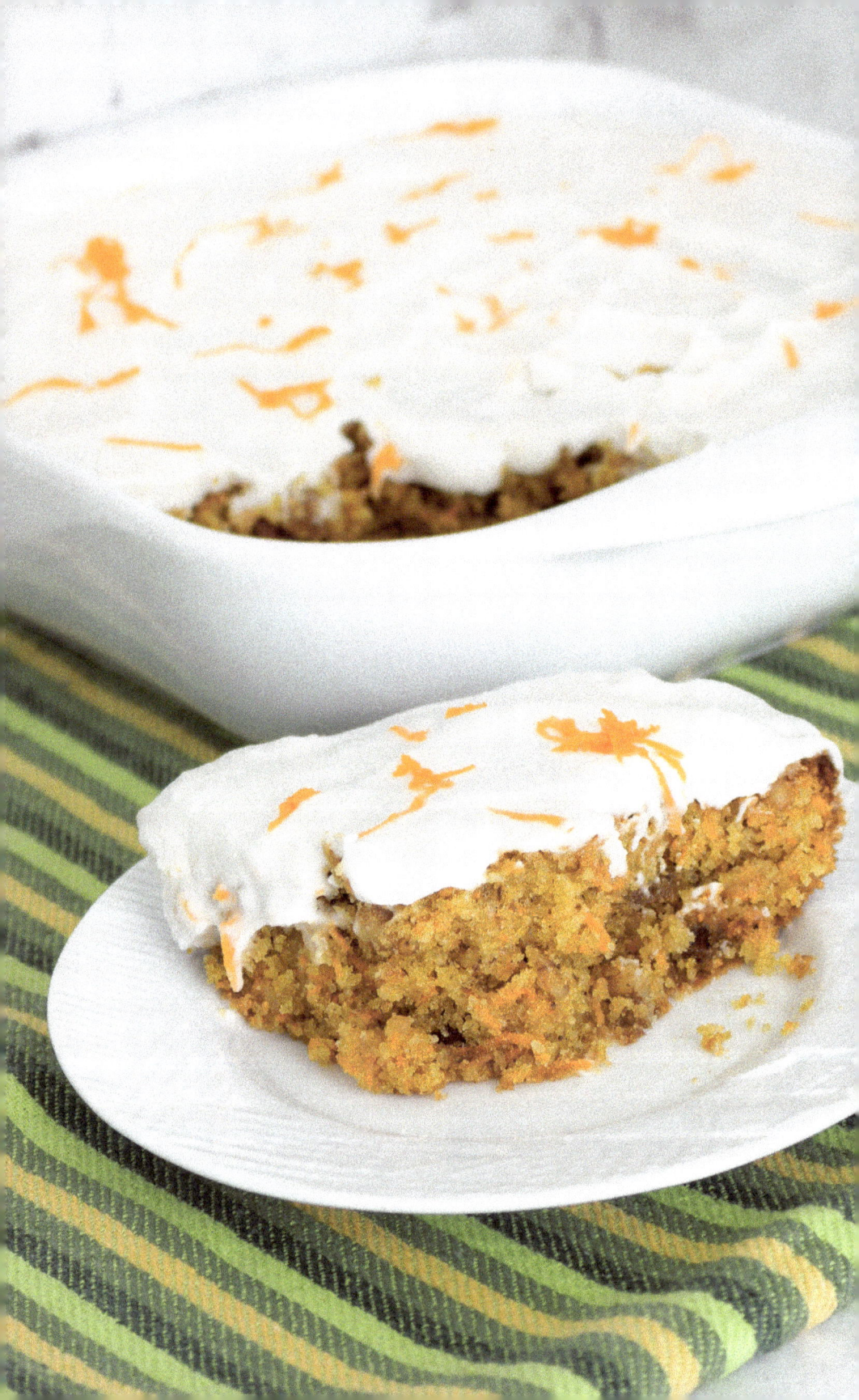

Carrot Walnut and Raisin Cake

TIME: 30 MINUTES | MAKES: 16 SQUARES (2-INCH X 2-INCH)

Ingredients

- 2 large eggs
- 3/4 cup (135 grams) brown sugar
- 1/2 cup (95 grams) seed oil
- 1 1/2 (160 grams) almond meal
- 1/2 cup (50 grams) oat flour
- 1/4 teaspoon (1 gram) baking soda
- 1/4 teaspoon (1 gram) baking powder
- 1/4 teaspoon (1 gram) salt
- 1/4 teaspoon (1 gram) allspice
- 1 cup (110 grams) finely grated carrots
- 1/3 cup (45 grams) raisins, coarsely chopped if preferred
- 1/2 cup (50 grams) walnuts, coarsely chopped

Frosting (optional)

- 2 – 3 cups can coconut cream, refrigerate
- 1 tablespoon maple syrup
- 1 teaspoon vanilla extract

Instructions

1. Preheat oven at 350F (180C). Grease and flour 8-inch square baking pan
2. In a large mixing bowl, combine the eggs, sugar and oil. Combine the almond meal, baking soda, baking powder, salt and allspice. Stir in carrots, raisins and walnuts
3. Pour into greased baking pan. Bake 30 – 35 minutes or until a toothpick inserted near the centre comes out clean. Cool for 10 minutes before removing from pan to wire rack to cool completely
4. For frosting, in another bowl, beat in coconut cream, maple syrup and vanilla until achieved desired consistency. Spread frosting over square. Serve and enjoy

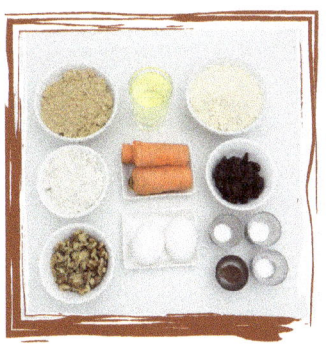

VEGETARIAN

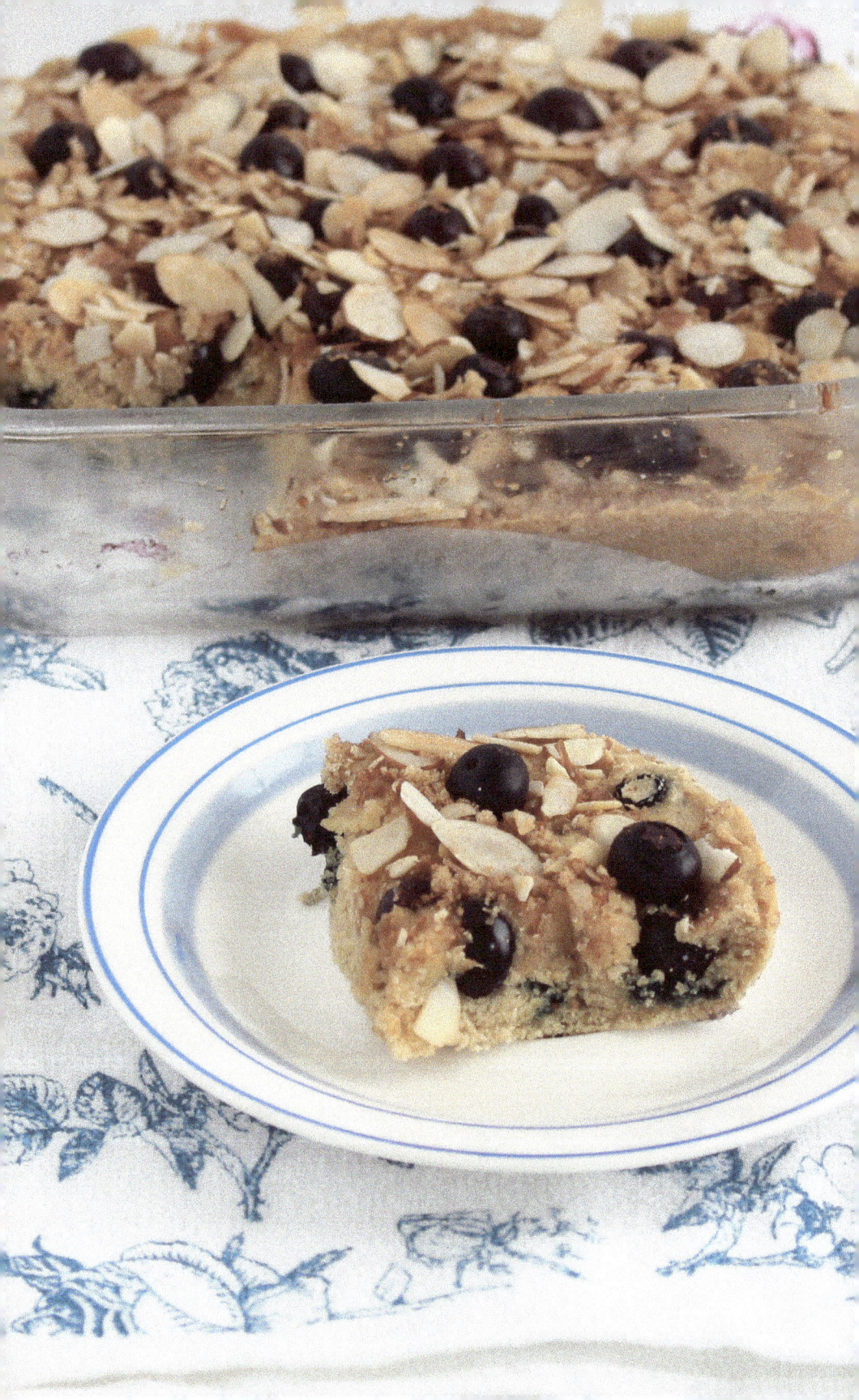

Blueberry Almond Coffee Cake

TIME: 30 MINUTES | MAKES: 8-INCH SQUARE

Ingredients

- 1 cup (160 grams) cassava flour
- 3/4 cup (140 grams) brown sugar
- 1 teaspoon (4 grams) baking powder
- 1/4 teaspoon (2 grams) baking soda
- 1/4 teaspoon (1 gram) salt
- 1 large egg
- 2/3 cup (145 grams) non-dairy milk
- 2 tablespoons (24 grams) butter, melted and cooled
- 1 tablespoon (10 grams) lemon juice
- 1/2 teaspoon (1 gram) almond extract
- 1 cup (145 grams) fresh blueberries

Topping
- 1/3 cup (50 grams) blueberries
- 1/2 cup (40 grams) sliced almonds
- 1 tablespoon (12 grams) brown sugar
- 1/4 teaspoon ground cinnamon

Instructions

1. Preheat the oven to 350F (180C). Grease an 8-inch square baking dish. or line with parchment paper.
2. In a large bowl combine almond meal, sugar, baking powder, baking soda and salt; Mix to combine.
3. In a medium bowl, whisk the egg, non-dairy milk, butter, lemon juice and almond extract. Add the almond meal mixture and stir until combined. Add blueberries and gently fold in batter. Pour into prepared baking dish.
4. Topping: top with blueberries. Combine the almonds, brown sugar and cinnamon, sprinkle over the top.
5. Bake 25 – 30 minutes, or until a toothpick inserted near the centre comes out clean. Cool on a wire rack. Serve and enjoy!

GRAIN-FREE | PALEO | VEGETARIAN

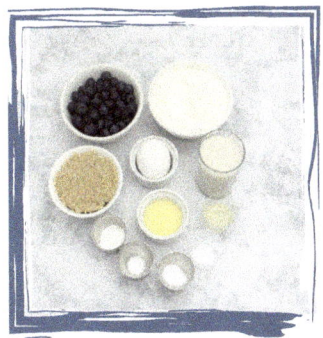

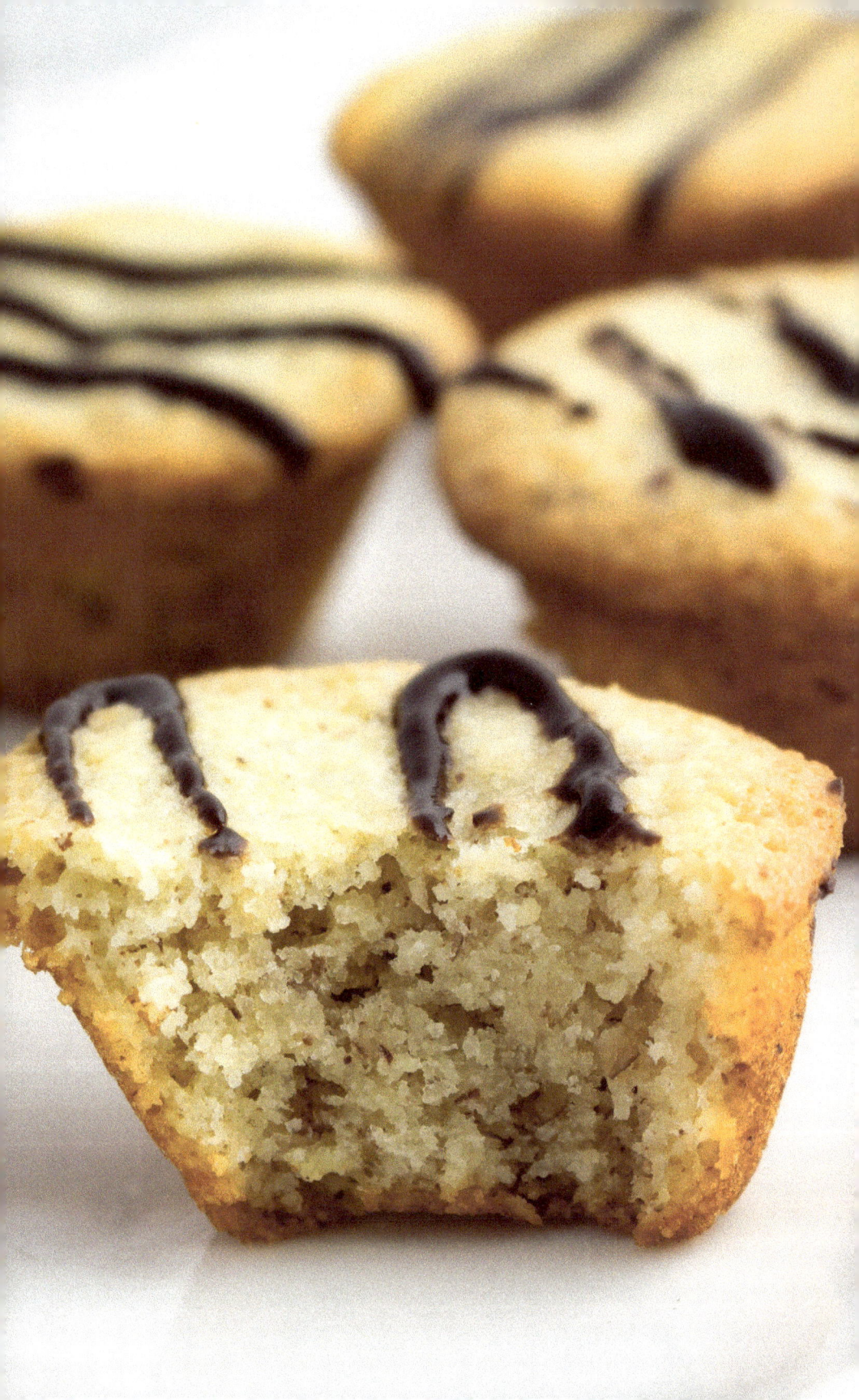

Almond Pecan Mini Cupcakes

TIME: 12 MINUTES | MAKES: 24 CUPCAKES

Ingredients

- 1-1/2 cups (140 grams) almond meal
- 1/2 teaspoon (1 gram) baking powder
- 1/8 teaspoon salt
- 2 large eggs
- 1/2 cup (95 grams) sugar
- 1/3 cup vegan butter, melted, and cooled
- 1/2 cup finely chopped pecans

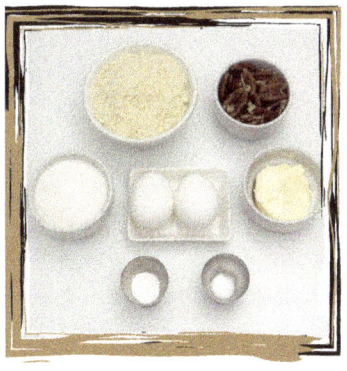

Instructions

1. Preheat the oven at 400F (180C). Grease or line mini muffin pan for 18 cupcakes.
2. In medium bowl, combine the almond meal, baking powder, and salt. Set aside.
3. In a large bowl, add the eggs and sugar; beat with an electric mixer until pale and thick. Add the butter and beat until well combined. Add the almond meal mixture in 2 batches and beat after each batch. Gently stir in pecans.
4. Spoon batter into baking pan until each cup is about 3/4 full. Bake in oven for 10 – 12 minutes until risen and golden. Let the cupcakes cool in the pan for 5 minutes, then transfer to wire rack to cool completely. Serve and enjoy with your choice of frosting if desired.

GRAIN-FREE | VEGETARIAN

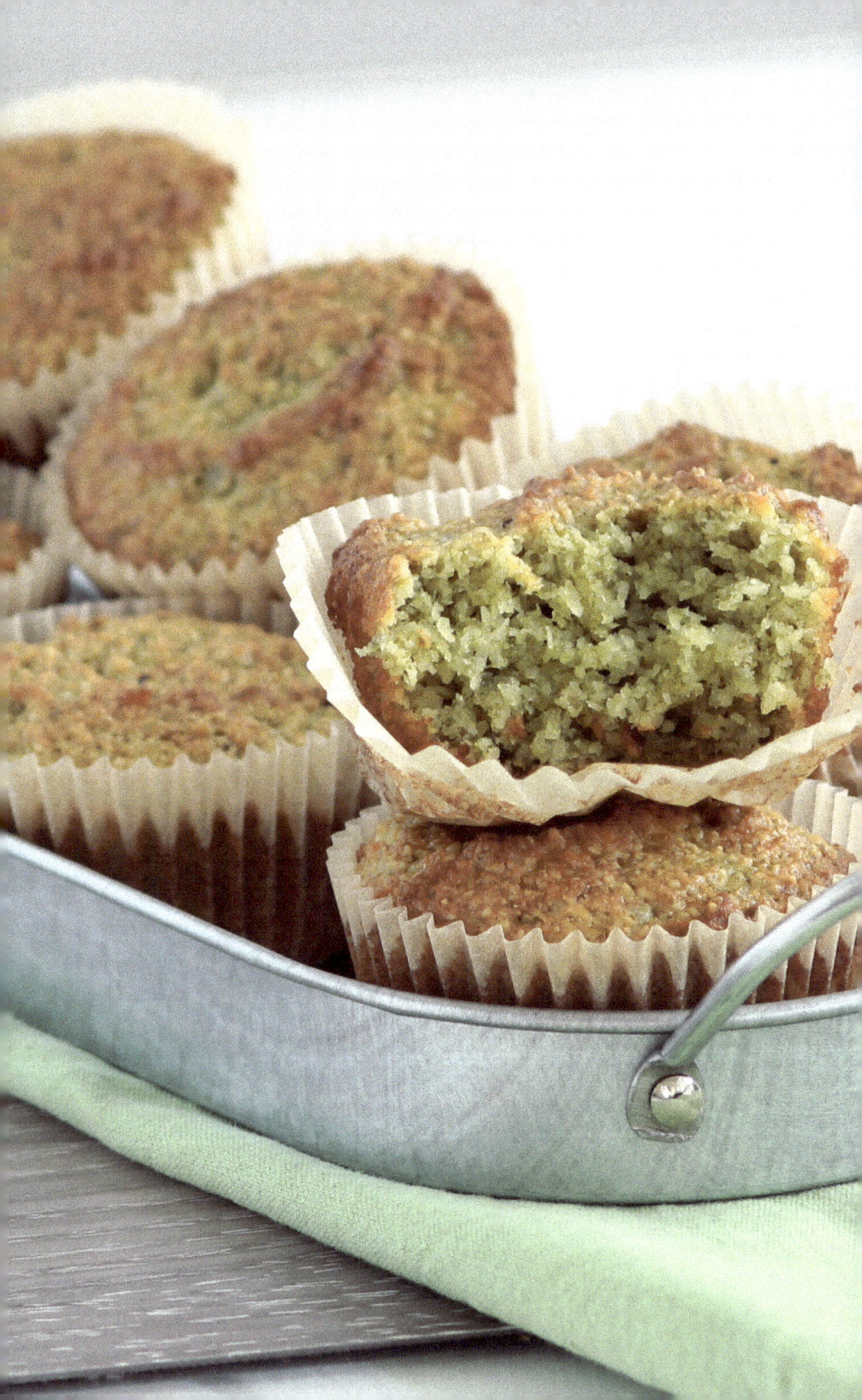

Pumpkin Seed Coconut Kiwi Cupcakes

TIME: 20 MINUTES | MAKES: 18 CUPCAKES

Ingredients

- 2 cups (280 grams) pumpkin seeds, finely grounded
- 1-1/2 cups (115 grams) finely shredded dried coconut
- 1/2 cup (105 grams) organic sugar
- 2 teaspoons (10 grams) baking powder
- 4 (250 grams) kiwi, ripe
- 3 large eggs
- 1/4 cup (55 grams) canola oil

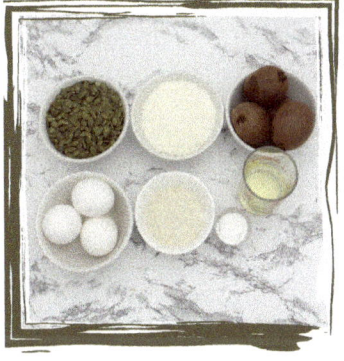

Instructions

1. Preheat the oven to 400F (200C). Grease muffin pan or line with muffin paper liners.
2. In medium bowl combine ground pumpkin seeds, shredded coconut, sugar, and baking powder; Mix to combine. Set aside.
3. In a food processor, add the kiwi and puree. Set aside.
4. In a large bowl, whisk the eggs and the oil. Add the kiwi mixture and whisk to combine. Add the pumpkin seed mixture and stir gently until combined.
5. Scoop or use a 1/3 cup measure to add batter to muffin pan. Bake 20 minutes, until risen, golden brown and firm to the touch. Remove from oven and let cool in pan for 5 minutes. Then transfer to a wire rack to finish cooling. Serve and enjoy!

GRAIN-FREE | PALEO | VEGETARIAN

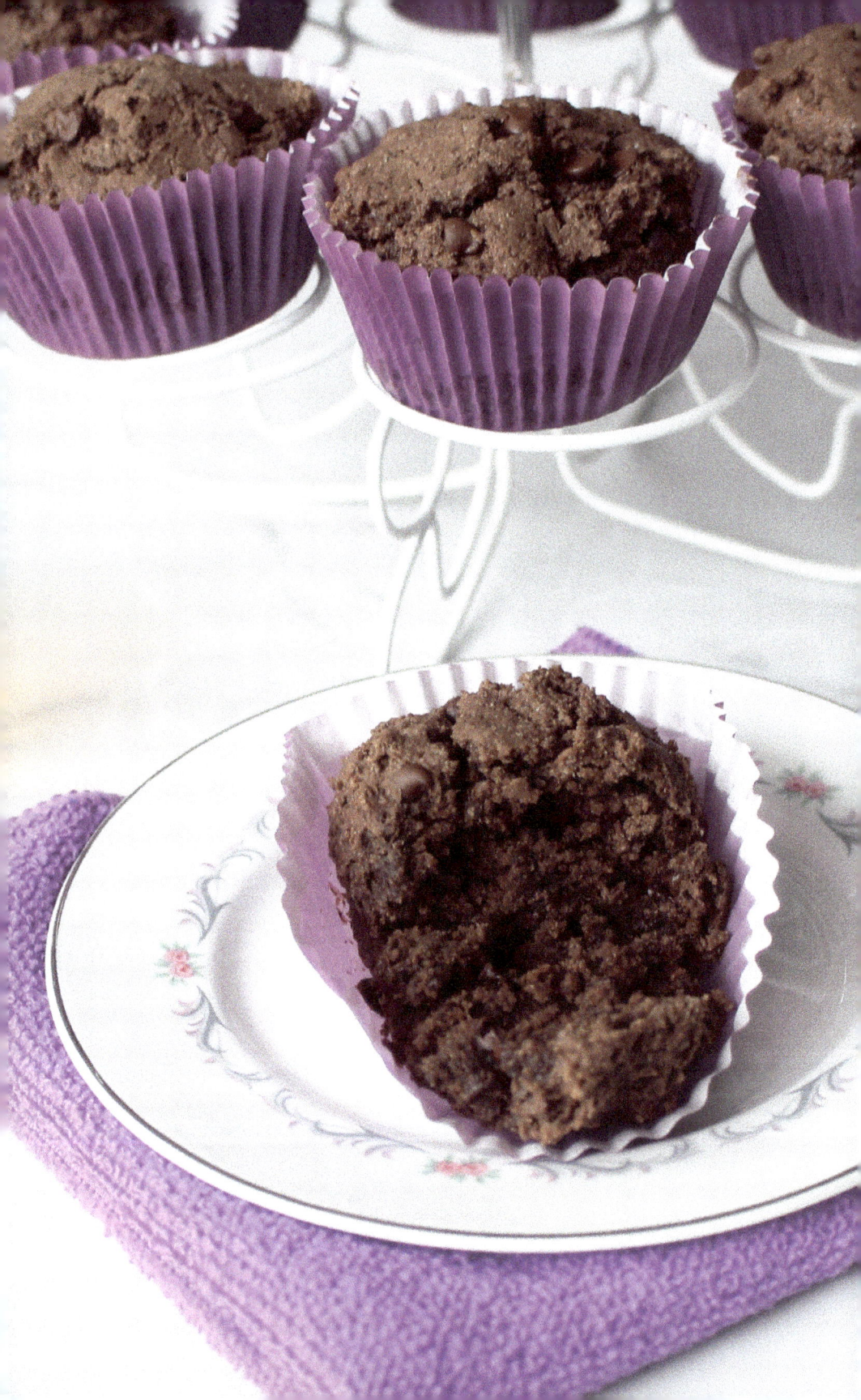

Double Chocolate and Black Bean Cupcakes

TIME: 20 MINUTES | MAKES: 12 CUPCAKES

Ingredients

- 1 1/3 cups (130 grams) oat flour
- 1/3 cup (30 grams) cocoa powder
- 1/2 cup (75 grams) brown sugar
- 1 tablespoon (12 grams) baking powder
- 1/4 teaspoon salt
- 2 large eggs
- 1/3 cup (60 grams) vegetable or seed oil
- 1 cup (170 grams) canned black beans, drained and rinsed
- 1/2 cup (80 grams) mini-chocolate chips

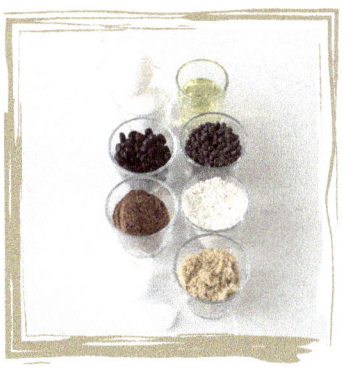

Instructions

1. Preheat oven at 350F (180C). Grease a 12-cup muffin pan or line with muffin paper liners.
2. In a large bowl, sift together the oat flour and cocoa powder, stir in the sugar, baking powder and salt. Make sure to have no lumps from the brown sugar. Make a well in centre.
3. In a medium bowl, lightly whisk the eggs, set aside. In a blender or food processor, combined the oil and black beans until creamy add to the egg mixture and stir well. Pour into the centre of the dry mixture. Add the chocolate chips, stir gently until just combined; do not over mix.
4. Spoon into muffin cups to 3/4 full or use ice cream scoop to pour batter. Bake in the preheated oven for about 18 - 20 minutes, until risen and firm to the touch.
5. Let the cupcakes cool in the pan for 5 minutes, then transfer to wire rack and let cool completely.

VEGETARIAN

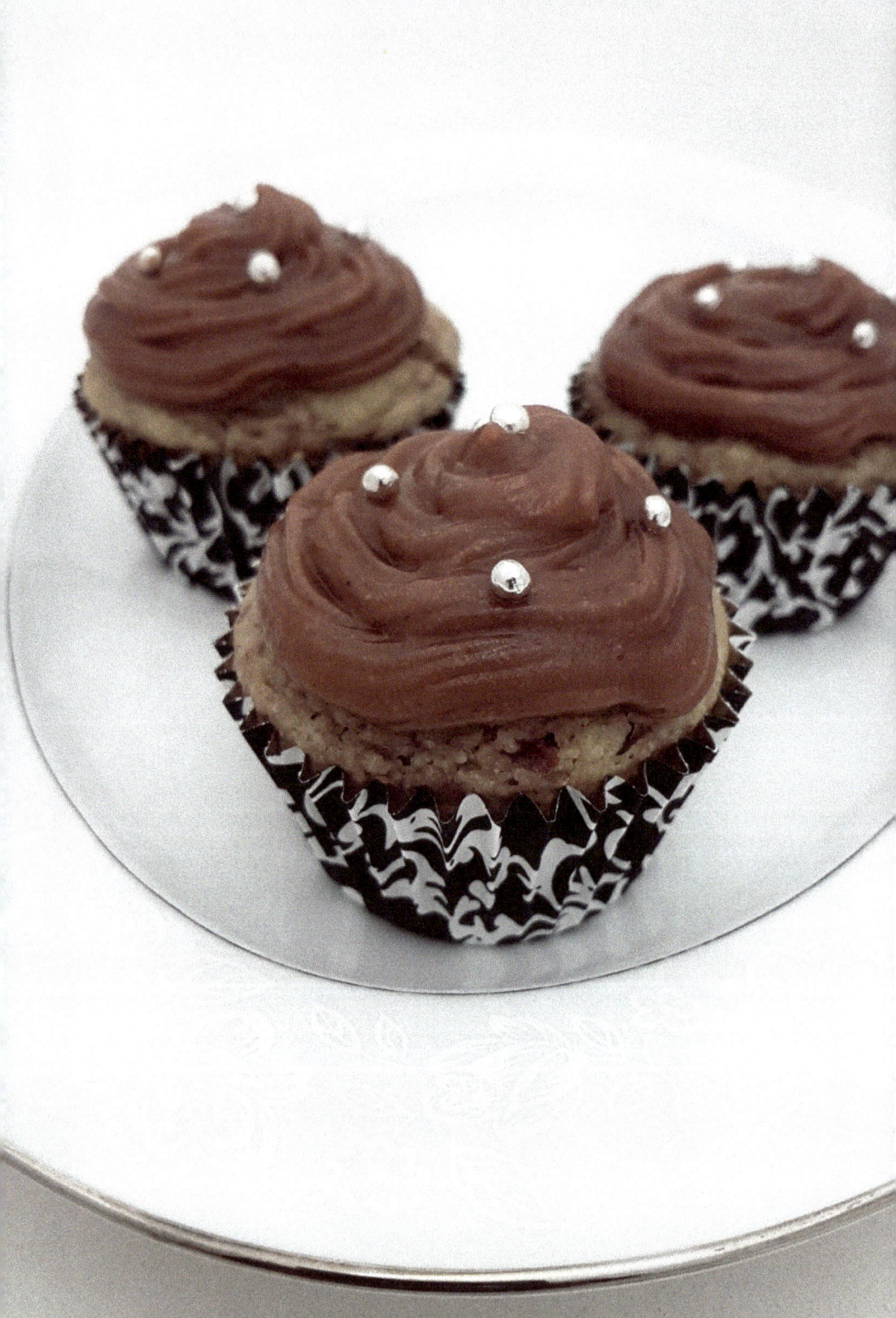

Raspberry Cupcake with Avocado Cranberry Frosting

TIME: 20 MINUTES | MAKES: 12 CUPCAKES

Ingredients

- 2 cups (200 grams) almond meal
- 3/4 cup (115 grams) buckwheat flour
- 1/2 cup (75 grams) brown sugar
- 1 tablespoon (12 grams) baking powder
- 1/4 teaspoon salt
- 2 large eggs
- 1 teaspoon (8 grams) vanilla extract
- 1/4 cup (65 grams) vegetable or seed oil
- 1/3 cup (70 grams) non-dairy milk
- 1/2 cup (70 grams) chopped fresh raspberries
- Avocado Cranberry Frosting
- 1 large avocado
- 1 cup (250 grams) canned jellied cranberries
- 1/4 cup (35 grams) brown sugar

Instructions

1. Preheat oven at 350F (180C). Grease a 12-cup muffin pan or line with muffin paper liners.
2. In a large bowl, whisk together the almond meal, buckwheat flour, sugar, baking powder and salt. Make sure to have no lumps from the brown sugar. Make a well in the centre. Set aside.
3. In a medium bowl, lightly whisk the egg, vanilla and oil, then whisk in the milk. Pour liquid mixture in the centre of the dry ingredients and beat with an electric mixer until combined. Fold in strawberries; do not over mix.
4. Spoon into muffin cups to 3/4 full or use ice cream scoop to pour batter. Bake in the preheated oven for about 15 - 20 minutes, until rise, golden brown and firm to the touch. Let the muffins cool in the pan for 5 minutes, then transfer to wire rack and let cool completely
5. To make frosting, in a blender or food processor, add the avocado, cranberries and sugar and process until smooth. Spread or pipe the frosting on cupcakes.

GRAIN-FREE | PALEO | VEGETARIAN

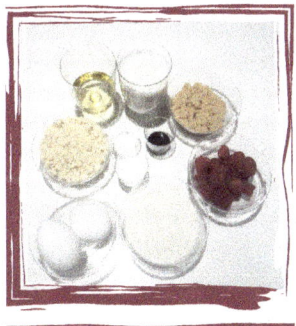
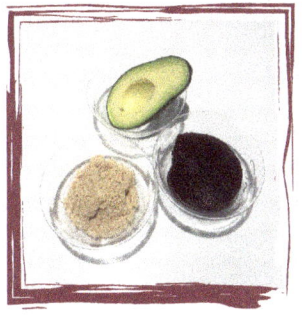

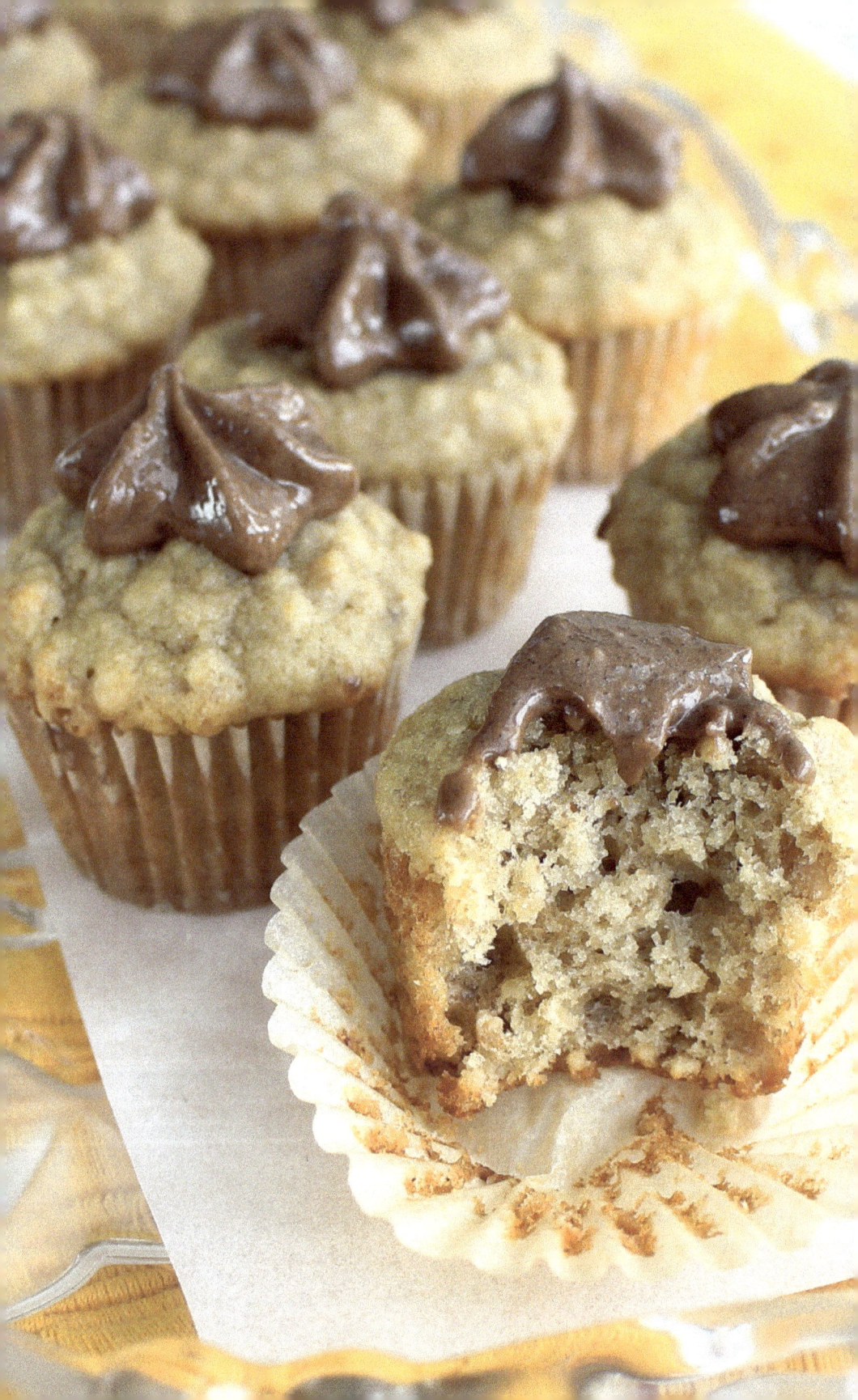

Peanut and Banana Mini Cupcakes

TIME: 20 MINUTES | MAKES: 36 CUPCAKES

Ingredients

- 2 cups (170 grams) oat flour
- 1-1/2 cups (215 grams) peanuts, unsalted
- 3/4 cup (100 grams) brown sugar
- 1 tablespoon (12 grams) baking powder
- 2 large eggs
- 1/4 cup (65 grams) vegan margarine or butter, melted and cooled
- 1-3/4 cups (330 grams) mashed overripe bananas (about 2 medium-size)

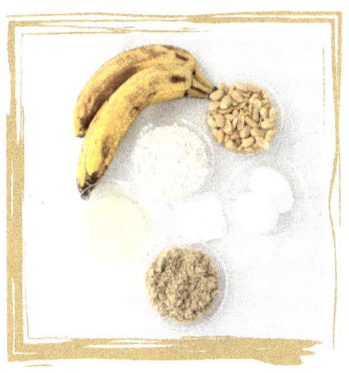

Instructions

1. Preheat oven to 350F (180C). Grease 36 cups of min-muffin pan or line with muffin paper liners.
2. Process peanuts in blender or food processor until finely grounded but not butter smooth. Set aside.
3. In a large bowl, combine the oat flour, sugar, and baking powder. Make sure to have no lumps from the brown sugar. Make a well in centre. Set aside.
4. In a medium bowl, lightly whisk the eggs, whisk in the butter and then stir in the mashed bananas. Pour liquid mixture into the centre of the dry mixture. Beat with an electric mixer until combined. Gently stir in peanuts; do not over mix.
5. Spoon or use a cookie scoop to pour batter 3/4 full into the prepared muffin pan. Bake for about 18 - 20 minutes, until risen and firm to the touch.
6. Let the cupcakes cool in the pan for 5 minutes, then transfer to wire rack and let cool completely.

Frosting (optional): mix 1 cup smooth peanut butter with 1/4 cup maple syrup and 2 to 4 tablespoons cocoa powder. Spread as desired.

VEGETARIAN

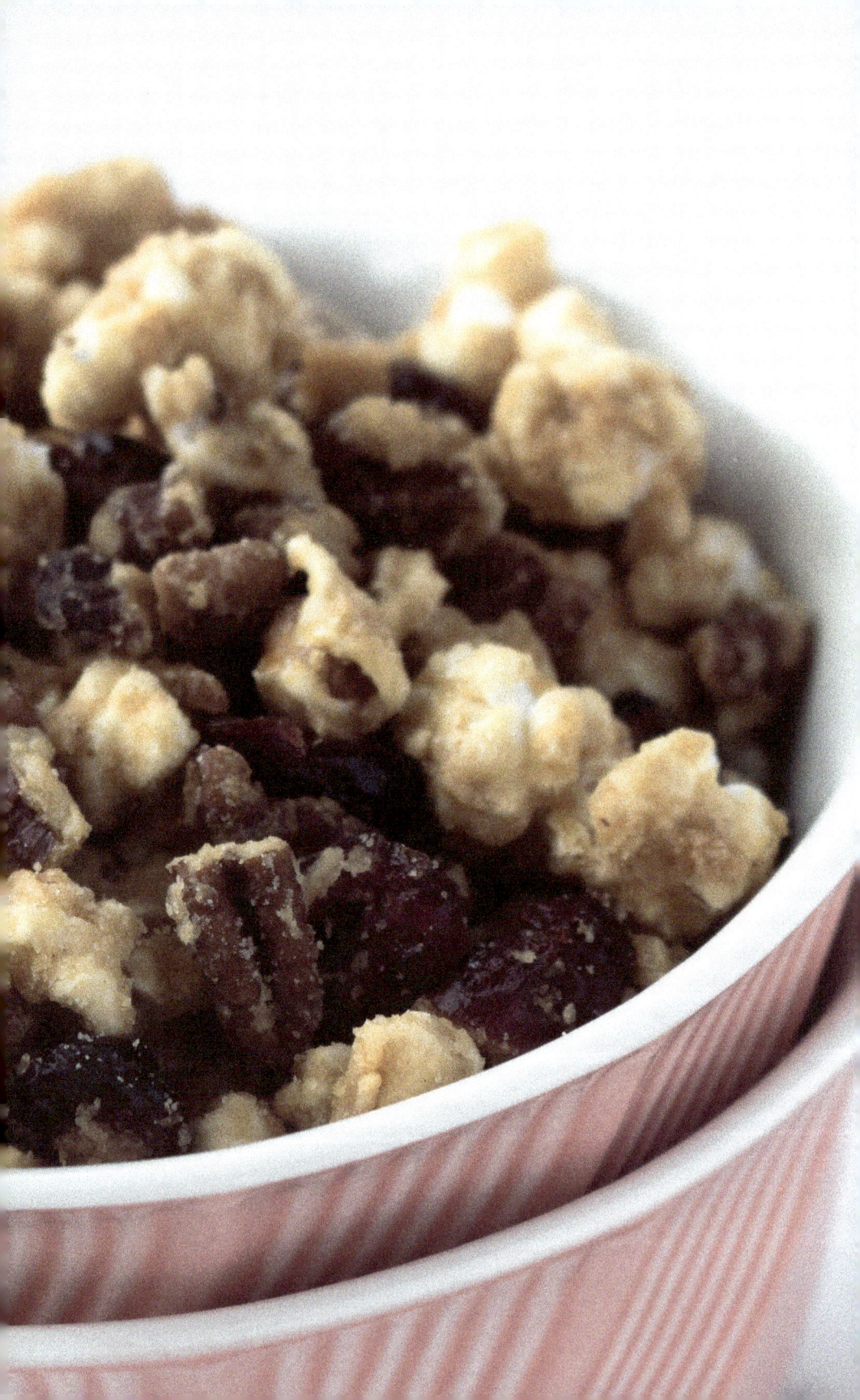

Caramel Pecan Cranberry Coconut Popcorn

TIME: 45 MINUTES | MAKES: 8 CUPS

Ingredients

- 1 bag of microwave popcorn (popped)
- 1 cup (105 grams) pecans, chopped
- 1/2 cup (30 grams) shredded coconut
- 1/2 cup (70 grams) dried cranberries
- 3/4 cup (150 grams) vegan butter
- 3/4 cup (130 grams) brown sugar
- 1/2 cup (140 grams) maple syrup
- 1/2 teaspoon (3 grams) salt
- 1/4 teaspoon (1 gram) baking soda
- 1/2 teaspoon (1 gram) vanilla extract

Instructions

1. Preheat oven at 250F (120C).
2. In a large bowl mix together the popped corn, pecans, coconut, and cranberries. Set aside
3. In a large saucepan on medium heat, add the butter, brown sugar, maple syrup and salt. Heat and stir until boiling. Boil without stirring for 5 minutes.
4. Stir in baking soda and vanilla. Remove from heat, add the popcorn mixture, and stir until all pieces is coated. Spread on a large ungrease shallow pan.
5. Bake for 45 minutes in prepared oven, stirring every 15 minutes. Cool thoroughly. Serve and enjoy!

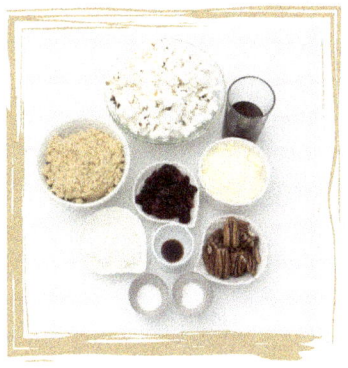

VEGAN | VEGETARIAN

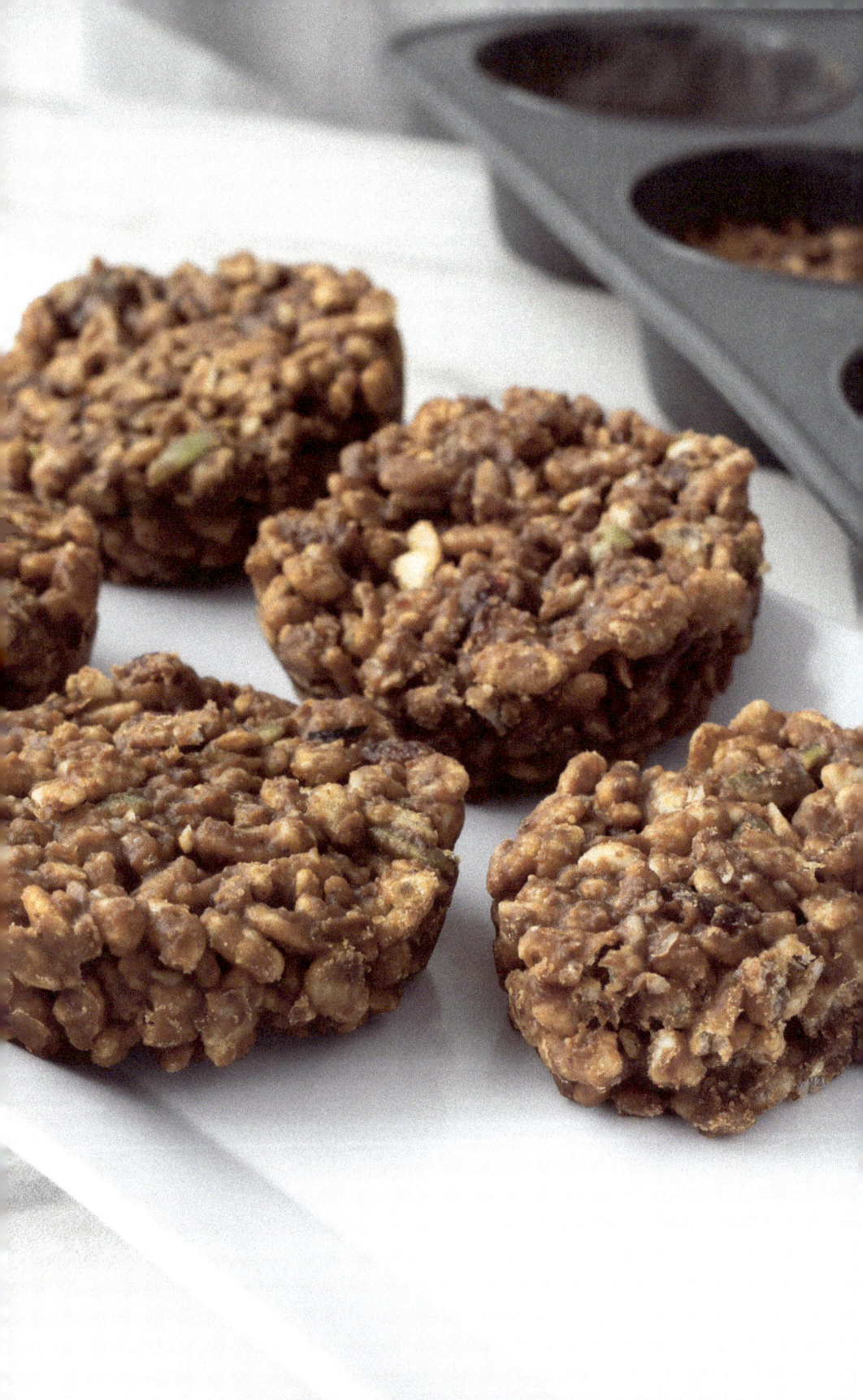

Brown Rice Crisp and Trail Mix Treats

TIME: 15 MINUTES | MAKES: 18 PIECES

Ingredients

- 4 cups (210 grams) brown rice crisp, vitamin D fortified
- 1 cup (145 grams) trail mix (dried fruits, nuts & seeds), coarsely grounded
- 3/4 cup (190 grams) almond butter
- 1/2 cup (150 grams) maple syrup
- 2 tablespoons (30 grams) coconut oil
- 1/2 cup (100 grams) vegan chocolate chips
- 1 teaspoon (5 grams) vanilla extract

Instructions

1. Greased an 8-inch square dish or desired silicone mold with oil.
2. In large bowl mix together the brown rice crisp and the trail mix. Set aside.
3. In a microwave-proof bowl, stir together the almond butter, maple syrup, coconut oil, and chocolate chips. Microwave on high for 30 seconds, stir and then microwave for additional 30 seconds or until chocolate chips is melted. Add the vanilla and stir until smooth.
4. Add the brown rice mixture and gently stir to combined. Add to baking dish or mold and press firmly. Cool in refrigerator for 30 or until cold and firm. Serve and enjoy!

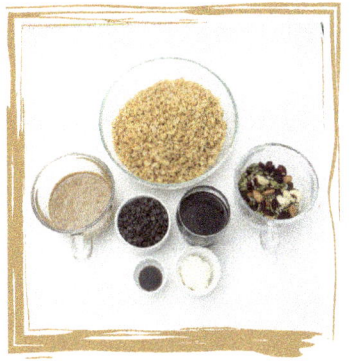

VEGAN | VEGETARIAN

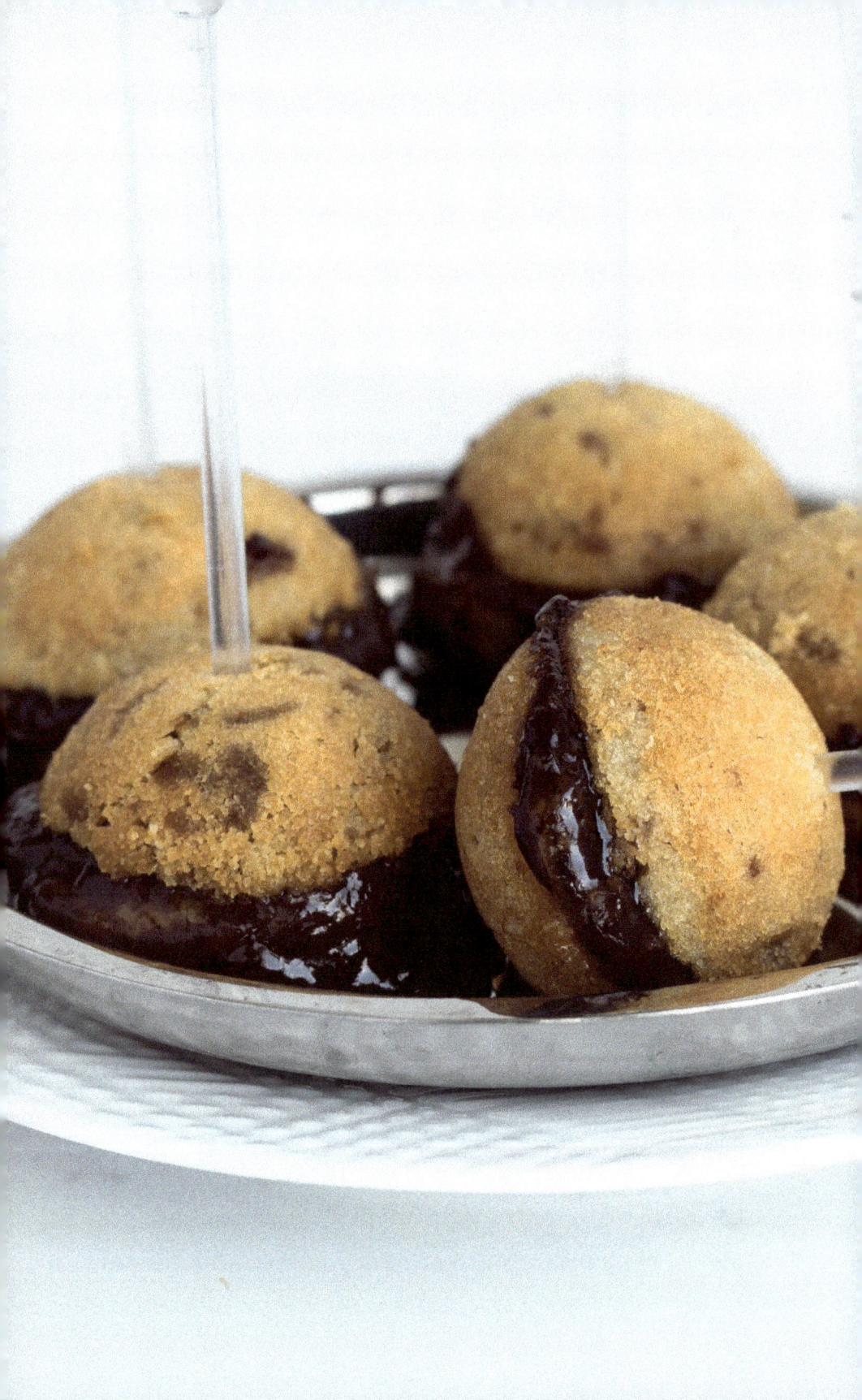

Fig Oat Mini Donuts

TIME: 20 MINUTES | MAKES: 15 PIECES

Ingredients

- 3/4 cup (90 grams) oat flour
- 1 teaspoon (4 grams) baking powder
- 1/4 teaspoon (1 gram) salt
- 1/3 cup (90 grams) rice milk, room temperature
- 2 tablespoons (40 grams) fig jam
- 2 tablespoons (24 grams) vegan butter, melted
- 1 teaspoon (3 grams) apple cider vinegar
- 1/4 cup (40 grams) dried figs, stem removed, finely chopped

Filling (optional)
- Fig jam and melted chocolate

Instructions

1. Preheat the oven at 350F (180C). grease donut pan.
2. In a large bowl, combine the oat flour, baking powder and salt. Add the rice milk, fig jam, butter, and apple cider vinegar. Stir well to combine. Stir in the dried figs.
3. For half-moon donuts, use a 1/2 tablespoon measure to pour batter into prepare donut pan. Bake 10 – 12 minutes, remove from oven and allow to cool for 5 minutes before transferring to a cooling rack.
4. For filling, add jam and then melted chocolate. Serve and enjoy!

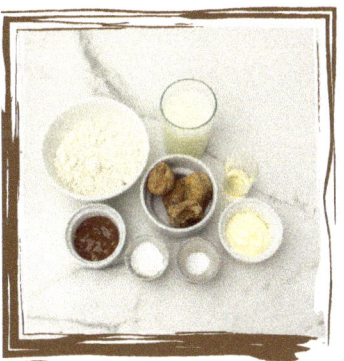

VEGAN | VEGETARIAN

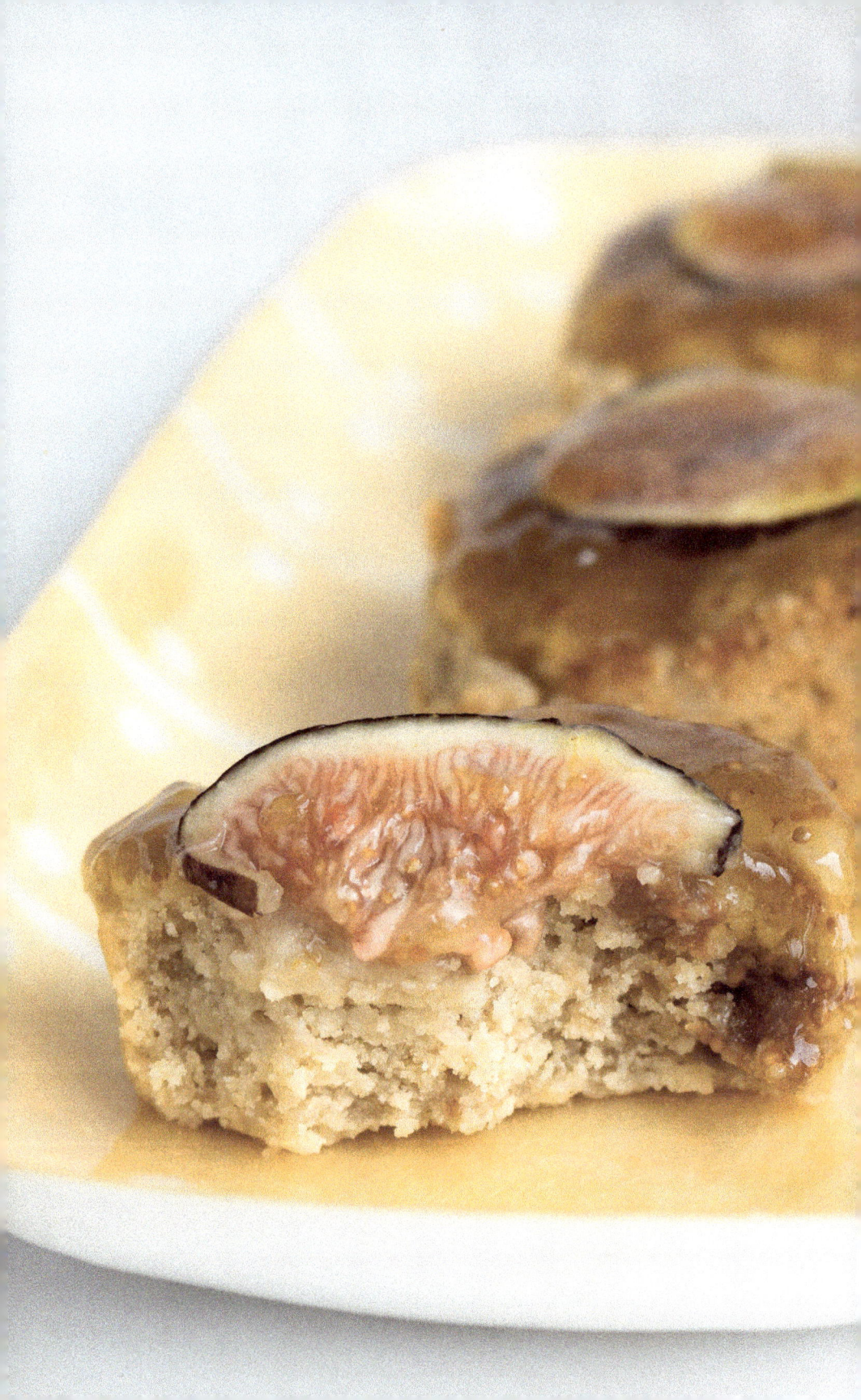

Fig Oat Scones

TIME: 20 MINUTES | MAKES: 12 PIECES

Ingredients

- 2 cups (200 grams) oat flour
- 1/2 cup (50 grams) brown sugar
- 2 teaspoons (8 grams) baking powder
- 1/4 teaspoon (1 gram) salt
- 1/4 cup (60 grams) cold vegan butter
- 1/2 cup dried figs, stem removed, finely chopped
- 1 cup (245 grams) dairy-free yogurt
- 1/2 teaspoon (2 grams) vanilla extract

Topping (optional)
- Fig Jam and sliced fresh figs

Instructions

1. Preheat the oven at 350F (180C). Line baking sheet with parchment paper or grease divided baking pan.
2. In a medium bowl, whisk together the oat flour, baking powder, and salt. Combine butter into flour mixture, using fork, pastry cutter, rub together with her hands. Mixture should resemble dry breadcrumbs. Stir in dried figs. Stir in yogurt and vanilla until mixture is evenly moist.
3. Divide batter using ice-cream scoop or 1/2 cup measuring cup onto prepared baking pan. Bake for 18 – 20 minutes or until edges of scones are golden brown and a wooden toothpick inserted in the centre comes out clean. Serve and enjoy!

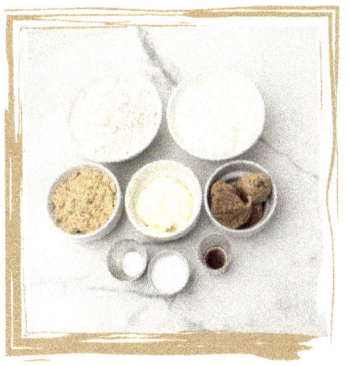

VEGAN | VEGETARIAN

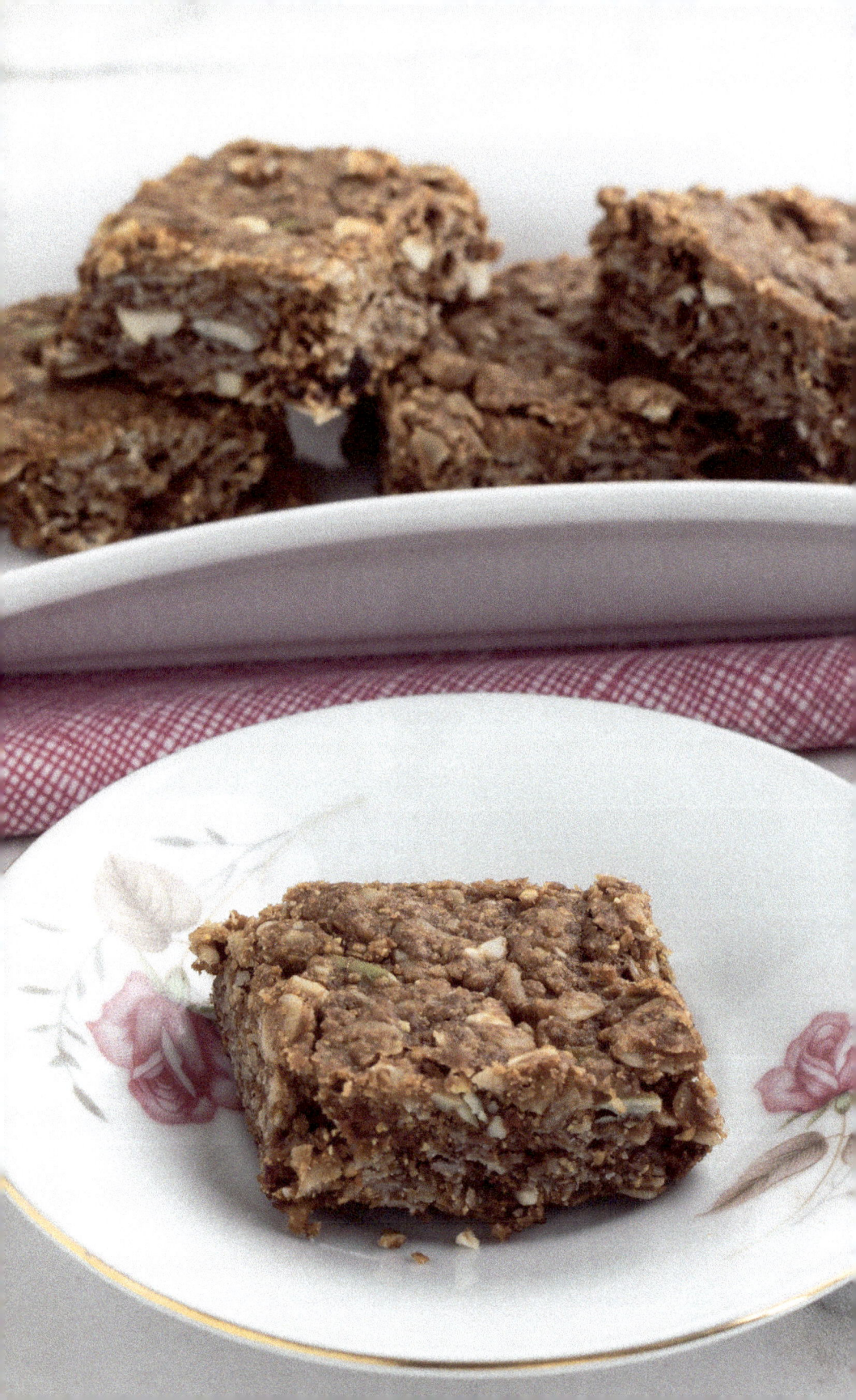

Pumpkin Seed Cranberry Mix Oat Squares

TIME: 15 MINUTES | MAKES: 18 SQUARES (2-INCH X 2-INCH)

Ingredients

- 2 cups (180 grams) rolled oats
- 1/3 cup (45 grams) ground flax seeds
- 1 teaspoon (4 grams) baking powder
- 1 cup (150 grams pkg) nuts-seeds-dried fruit mix
- 1/4 cup (60 grams) vegan butter, room temperature
- 1/2 cup (130 grams) almond butter
- 1/3 cup (55 grams) brown sugar
- 1/4 cup (65 grams) maple syrup
- 1/2 cup (70 grams) vegan chocolate pieces
- 1 teaspoon (4 grams) vanilla extract

Instructions

1. Preheat oven at 350F (180C). Grease a 9-inch or 8-inch square baking pan and line with parchment paper.
2. In a large bowl, combine the oats, flax seeds, and baking powder. In a food processor, finely chop the nut/fruit mix. Add to the oat mixture. Set a side.
3. In a large saucepan on medium heat, add the butter, almond butter, sugar, maple syrup, and chocolate chips. Heat gently, stirring occasionally, until the chocolate chips has melted. Remove from heat and stir in the vanilla. Add to the oat mixture and stir until combined.
4. Pour the batter into the prepared baking pan, pressing firmly to even out. Bake for 15 minutes, or until pale golden. Remove from oven, let cool in pan for 5 – 7 minutes before cutting into squares. Serve and enjoy!

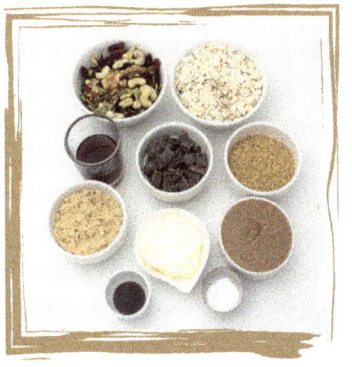

VEGAN | VEGETARIAN

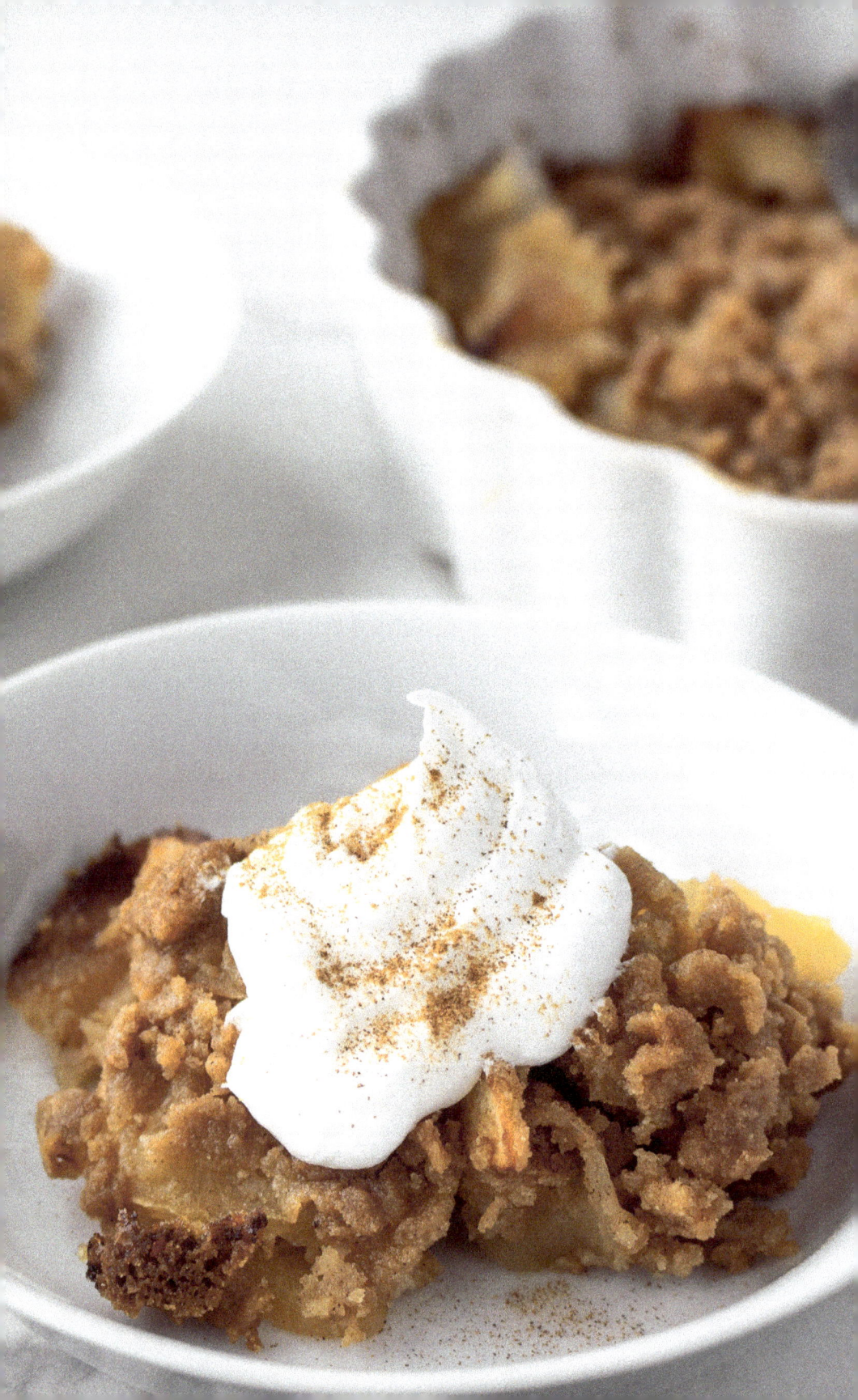

Apple Betty

TIME: 45 MINUTES | MAKES: 9-INCH PIE

Ingredients

- 2 cups (230 grams) sliced pared apples
- 2 tablespoons (40 grams) lemon juice
- 1/3 cup (65 grams) brown sugar
- 2/3 cups (80 grams) oat flour
- 1/4 teaspoon (1 gram) cinnamon
- 1/8 teaspoon nutmeg
- 3 tablespoons (40 grams) vegan butter

Instructions

1. Preheat oven at 375F (190C). Grease a 9-inch baking dish.
2. In a medium bowl, combine apples and lemon juice.
3. In a small bowl, combine sugar, oat flour, cinnamon, and nutmeg. Add the butter and rub it in with your fingertips or with a fork until the mixture looks like fine breadcrumbs.
4. Apple Betty is known for layers. Layer half the apples, then half the crumble, add next layer of apples and ending with crumble.
5. Bake in preheated oven for 45 minutes or until apples are tender and topping crisp. Serve and enjoy!

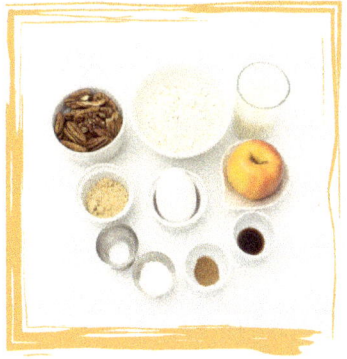

VEGAN | VEGETARIAN

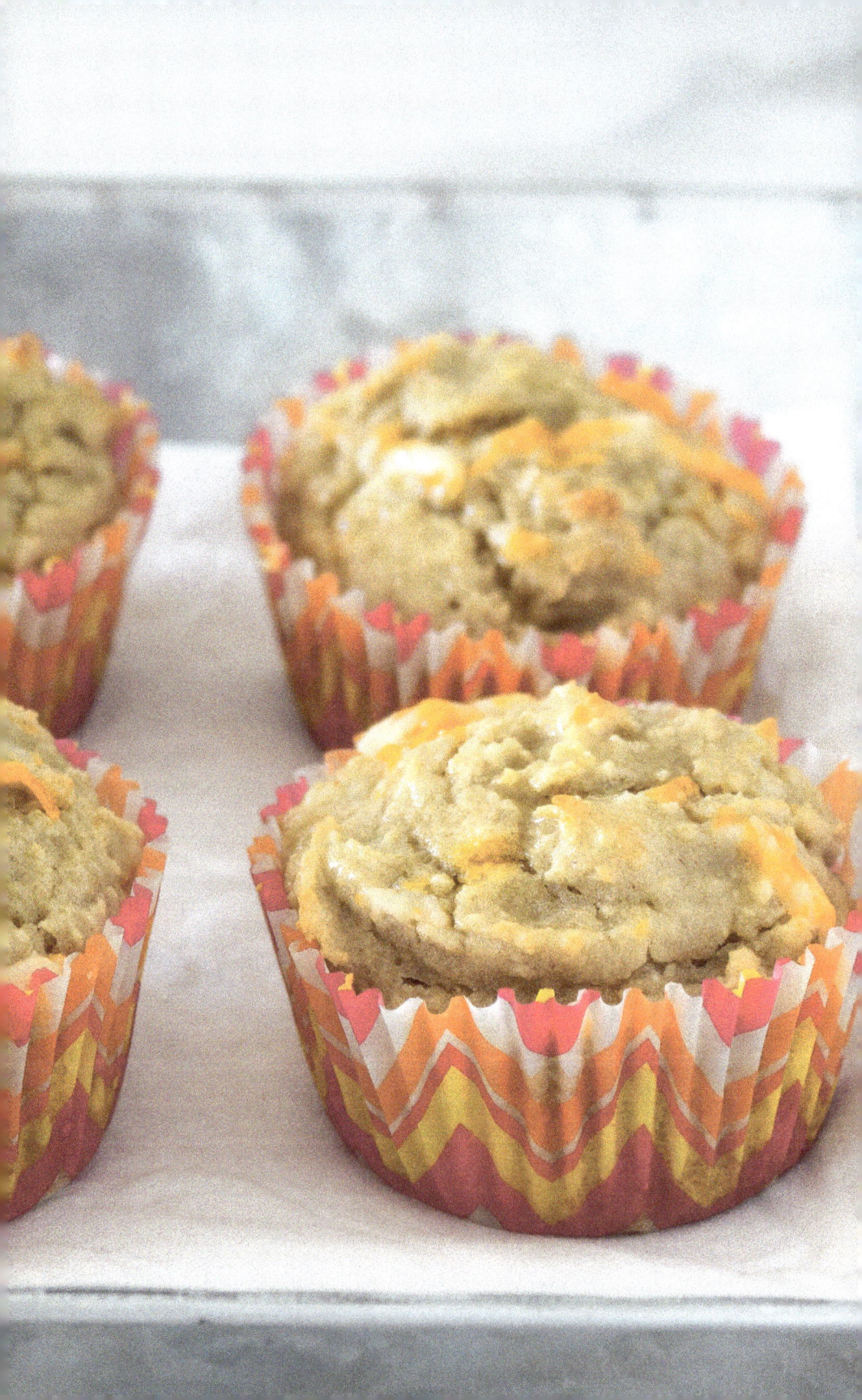

Potato Oat and Cheese Muffins

TIME: 20 MINUTES | MAKES: 12 MUFFINS

Ingredients

- 300 grams baking or russet potato
- 1 3/4 cups (165 grams) oat flour
- 1 tablespoon (10 grams) brown sugar
- 1 tablespoon (15 grams) baking powder
- 1/2 teaspoon (2 grams) baking soda
- 1/2 teaspoon (2 grams) salt
- 2 large eggs
- 3/4 cup (180 grams) rice milk
- 2 tablespoons (30 grams) vegan butter, melted
- 1 tablespoon (11 grams) apple cider vinegar
- 1/2 cup (35 grams) grated goat cheese

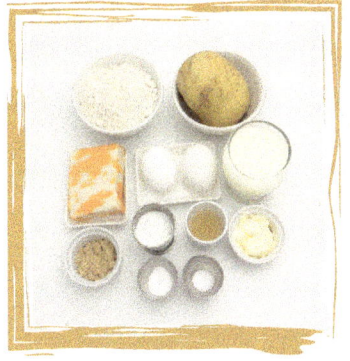

Instructions

1. Preheat oven to 375F (190C). Line with parchment paper or grease 12-cup muffin baking pan.
2. Scrub the potatoes well with a brush under running water. Then, pat them dry. Use a fork to poke holes all over the potato, about 5 times each. Wrap fully in paper towel and place in microwave. Cook for 3 minutes, flip the potatoes over, cook for another 3 minutes. Check for doneness. Using a fork to easily pierce into the potatoes when done. Set aside.
3. In a large bowl, combine the oat flour, sugar, baking powder, baking soda, and salt. Stir. Make well in centre.
4. Peel potato. In a medium bowl, mash potato. Add eggs, rice milk, butter, and apple cider vinegar. Beat with a whisk. Add to the centre of the flour mixture. Stir until just moistened. Fill muffin pan.
5. Bake for 18 to 20 minutes or until wooden toothpick inserted in centre of muffin comes out clean. Let stand in pan for 5 minutes before removing to wire rack to cool. Serve and enjoy!

VEGETARIAN

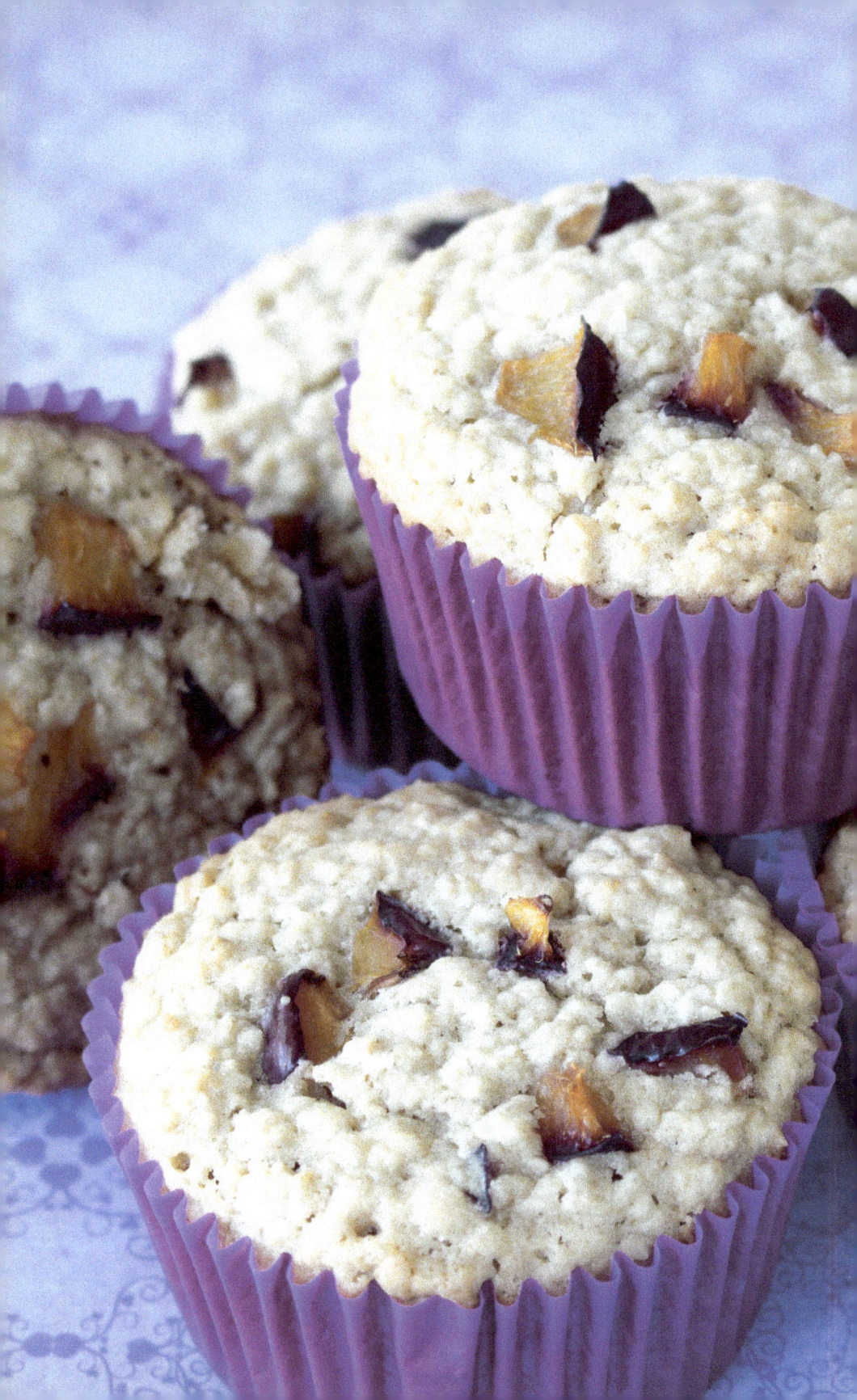

Prune Plum and Oat Muffins

TIME: 20 MINUTES | MAKES: 12 MUFFINS

Ingredients

- 1 cup (90 grams) oat flour
- 1 tablespoon (14 grams) baking powder
- 1/2 cup (85 grams) brown sugar
- 2 cups (160 grams) quick oats
- 1 cup (160 grams) pitted prune plums, chopped small (reserved 1/4 cup for topping)
- 2 large eggs
- 3/4 cup (180 grams) non-dairy milk (recipe – almond milk)
- 1/3 cup (65 grams) seed or vegetable oil
- 1 teaspoon (3 grams) vanilla extract

Instructions

1. Preheat oven to 375F (190C). Grease a 12-cup muffin pan or line with 12 muffin paper liners.
2. In a large bowl, sift together the oat flour and baking powder. Stir in the sugar, oats, and plums. Create a well in centre and set aside.
3. In a medium bowl, lightly beat the eggs, then beat the milk, oil, and vanilla. Pour the liquid in the well of the dry ingredients. Stir gently until just combined; do not over mix.
4. Use an ice-cream scoop or spoon the batter in the muffin pan. Bake for 20 minutes, until well risen, golden brown and firm to the touch.
5. Remove from oven and let muffins cool in pan for 5 minutes, then transfer to wire rack to finish cooling. Serve and enjoy!

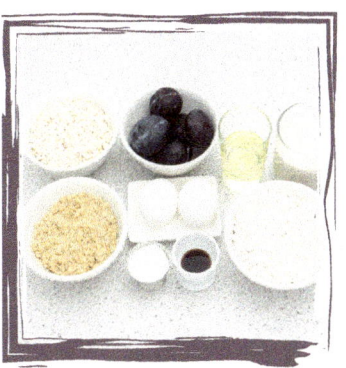

VEGETARIAN

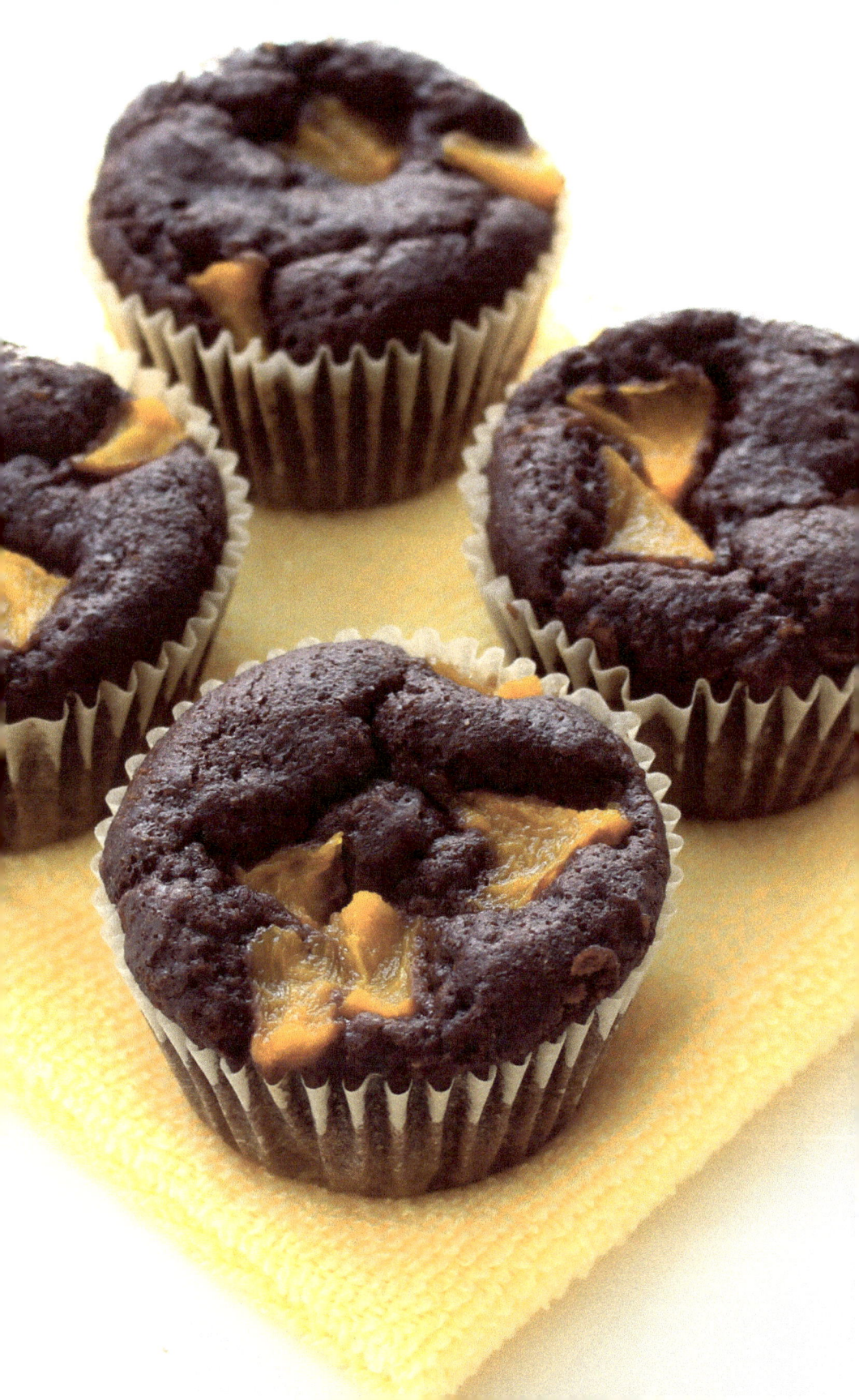

Vegan Chocolate Chickpea and Peach Muffins

TIME: 20 MINUTES | MAKES: 12 MUFFINS

Ingredients

- 1 1/2 cups (140) grams chickpea flour
- 1/2 cup (45 grams) cocoa powder
- 1/2 cup (75 grams) brown sugar
- 1 tablespoon (12 grams) baking powder
- 1/8 teaspoon salt
- 1/4 cup (65 grams) maple syrup
- 1/3 cup (80 grams) vegan margarine or butter, melted and cooled
- 1 cup (220) grams canned peaches, drained, chopped finely

Instructions

1. Place oven rack in middle of oven and then preheat oven to 350F (180C). Grease a 12-cup muffin pan or line with muffin paper liners.
2. In a large bowl, sift together the chickpea flour and coco powder, add the sugar, baking powder and salt. Make sure to have no lumps from the brown sugar. Make a well in centre.
3. In a medium bowl, whisk maple syrup and butter until creamy and then stir in peaches. Pour into the centre of the dry mixture. Stir gently until just combined; do not over mix.
4. Spoon into muffin cups to 3/4 full or use ice cream scoop to pour batter into the prepared muffin pan. Bake in the preheated oven for about 15 - 20 minutes, until risen and firm to the touch.
5. Let the muffins cool in the pan for 5 minutes, then transfer to wire rack and let cool completely.

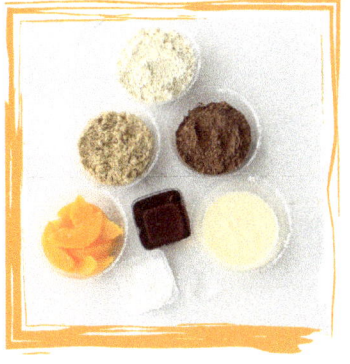

VEGETARIAN

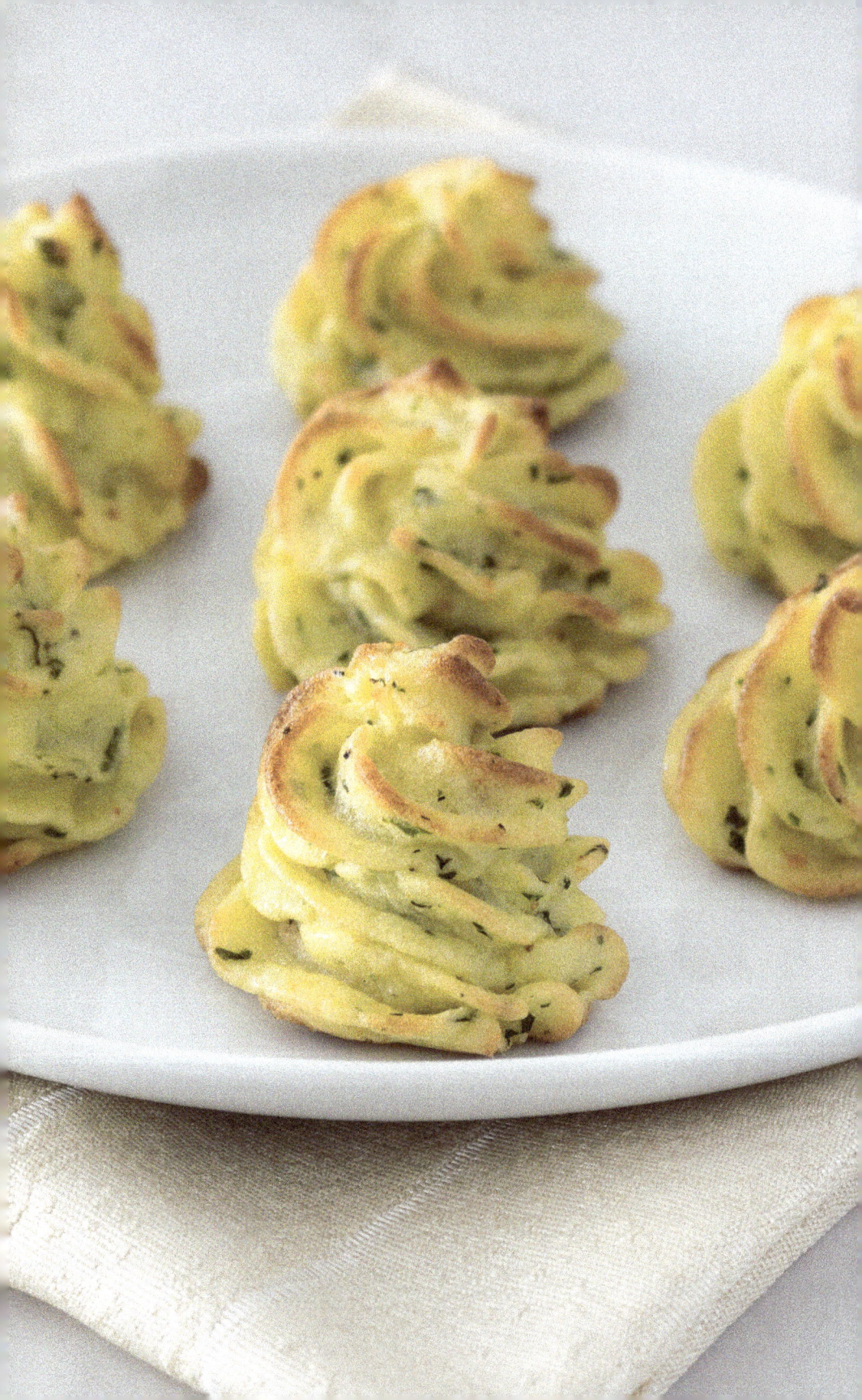

Duchess Potatoes with Kale

TIME: 20 MINUTES | MAKES: 24 PIECES

Ingredients

- 2 lbs. (970 grams) russet or baking potatoes, peeled, and quartered
- 3 large egg yolks
- 3 tablespoons (33 grams) non-dairy milk
- 2 tablespoons (22 grams) butter
- 1/2 teaspoon (2 grams) salt
- 1/2 teaspoon (1 gram) vegetable seasoning
- 1/4 cup (15 grams) finely chopped kale

Instructions

1. Place potatoes in a large saucepan and cover with water. Bring to a boil. Reduce heat; cover and simmer for 15 – 20 minutes or until tender. Drain.
2. Preheat oven to 425F (220C). Lined a baking sheet with parchment paper. In a large bowl, mashed the potatoes. Stir in the egg yolks, milk, butter, salt, vegetable seasoning, and kale until smooth.
3. Using a pastry bag or heavy-duty resealable plastic bag and a large star tip, pipe potatoes into large or small rounds on the baking sheet. Bake for 20 – 25 minutes or until golden brown. Cool on baking sheet for 5 minutes. Serve and enjoy!

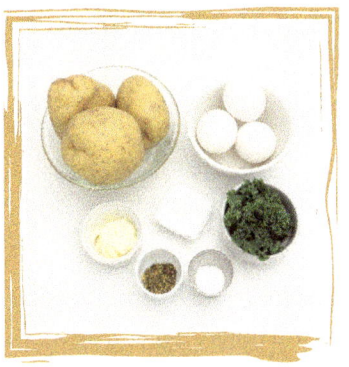

GRAIN-FREE | VEGETARIAN

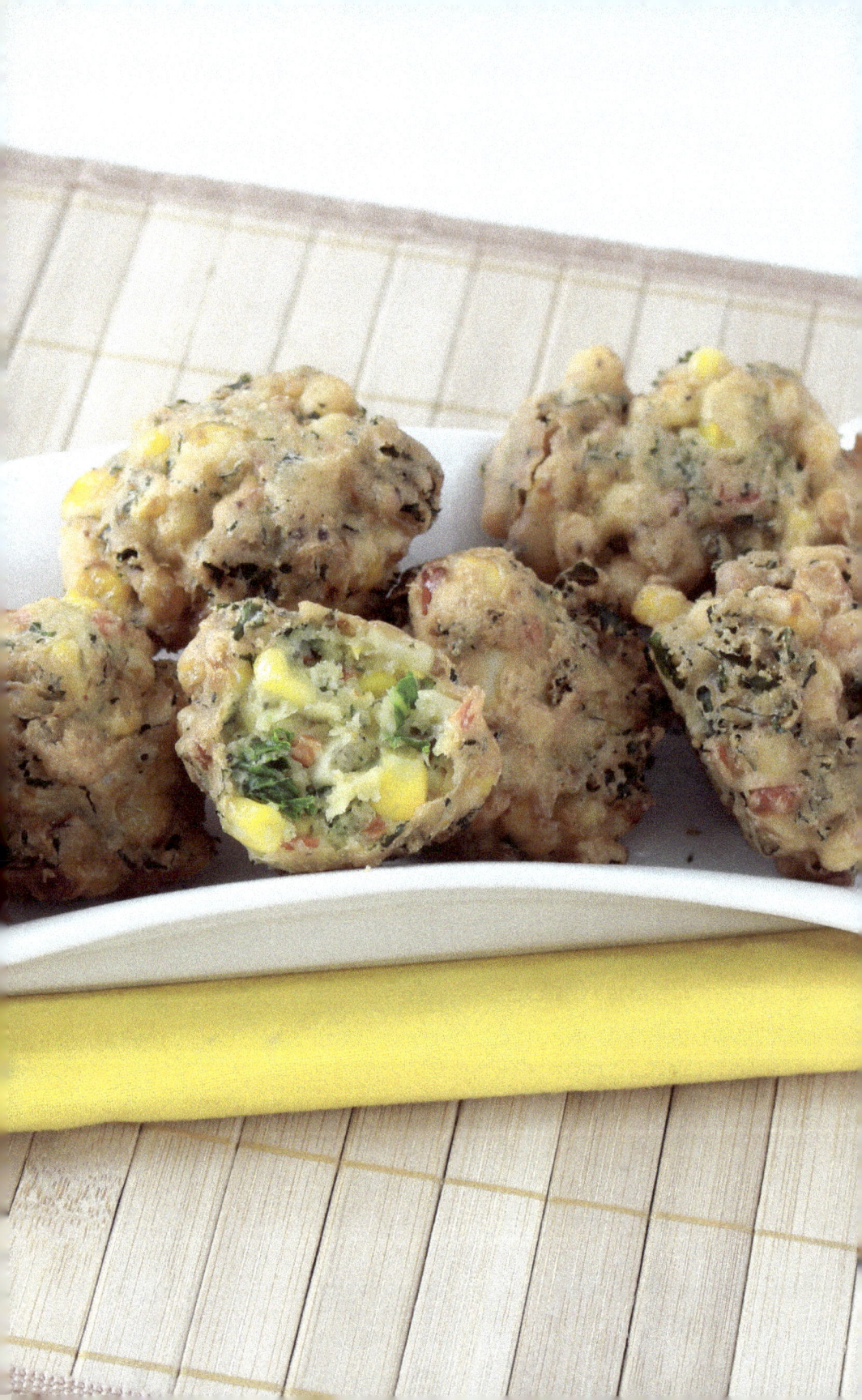

Corn Puffs with Kale and Bell Pepper

TIME: 15 MINUTES | MAKES: 12 PIECES

Ingredients

- 2 large eggs
- 1/4 cup (40 grams) vegetable oil
- 1 tablespoon (3 grams) vegetable seasoning
- 1/4 teaspoon salt (1 gram)
- 1/2 cup (55 grams) cassava flour
- 1 cup (150 grams) frozen corn, defrosted
- 1/2 cup (20 grams) finely chopped kale
- 1/4 cup (25 grams) finely chopped red bell pepper
- Oil for deep frying, if not baking

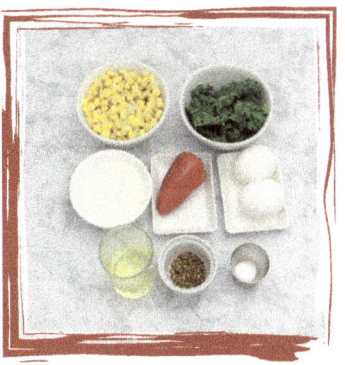

Instructions

1. Preheat the oven to 375F (190C). Grease mini muffin cups well.
2. In a large bowl, whisk the eggs, oil, vegetable seasoning and salt. Then whisk the cassava flour until combined. Stir the corn, kale and bell peppers into the batter
3. Use a small cookie scoop or one-tablespoon measure and divide batter into baking pan. Bake 15 minutes, until edges are golden brown around the edges. Remove from oven and let cool for 2 minutes. Then transfer to a wire rack to finish cooling.

NOTE: If deep frying – Fill deep saucepan or deep-fryer one-third full of oil and heat to 350F (180C). Scoop batter into oil and fry until golden brown. Drain on paper towels. Serve and enjoy with your favourite dipping sauce

GRAIN-FREE | VEGETARIAN

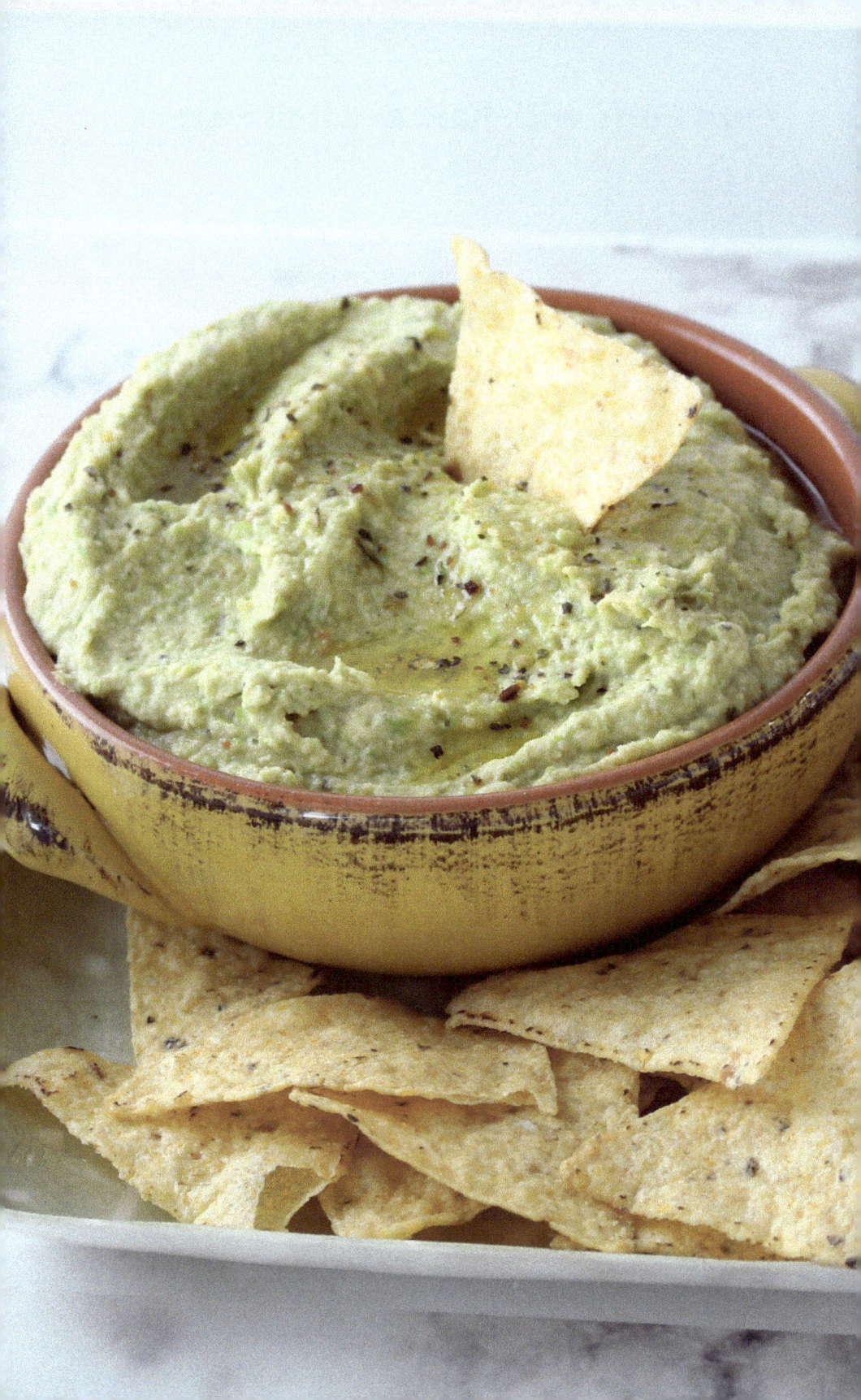

Asparagus Hummus

TIME: 15 MINUTES | MAKES: 3 CUPS

Ingredients

- 1/2 pound (230 grams) asparagus, cut into 1-inch pieces
- 2 cups (345 grams) can chickpeas, drained and rinsed
- 1/4 cup (45 grams) olive oil
- 2 tablespoons (18 grams) sesame tahini
- 1 tablespoon (8 grams) fresh lemon juice
- 2 teaspoons (6 grams) vegetable seasoning
- 1/2 teaspoon (2 grams) garlic powder
- Salt for desired taste (optional)

Instructions

1. Bring a large saucepan of water to boil over high heat. Prepare a bowl filled with ice water.
2. Add the asparagus pieces and cook until the asparagus into the ice water and set aside.
3. Drain and immediately add to the ice water stop cooking. Drain and transfer to a food processor. Add the chickpeas, oil, tahini, lemon juice, vegetable seasoning, and garlic powder. Process until the ingredients combined and smooth. Serve and enjoy!

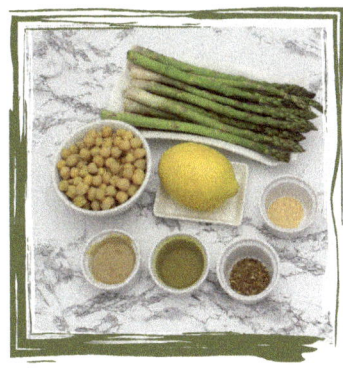

GRAIN-FREE | VEGETARIAN

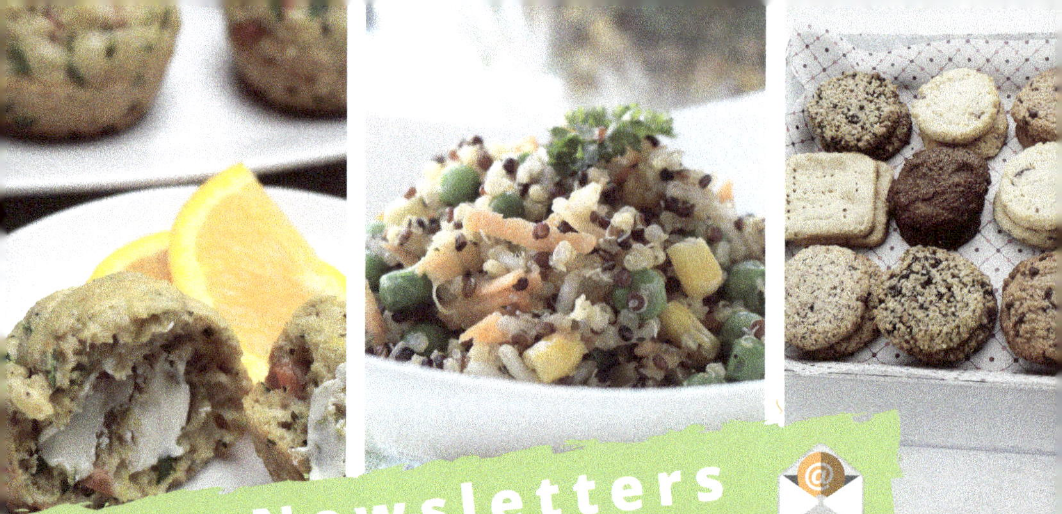

Newsletters

FREE Recipes in Your Inbox Every Week

- Delicious and nutritious recipes made from wholesome ingredients.
- Gluten-Free and Dairy-Free
- Cornstarch-Free and Yeast-Free.
- Breakfast, Lunch, Dinner and Snacks.

Magazines: Print & Online

www.eatforlifebymarsha.com

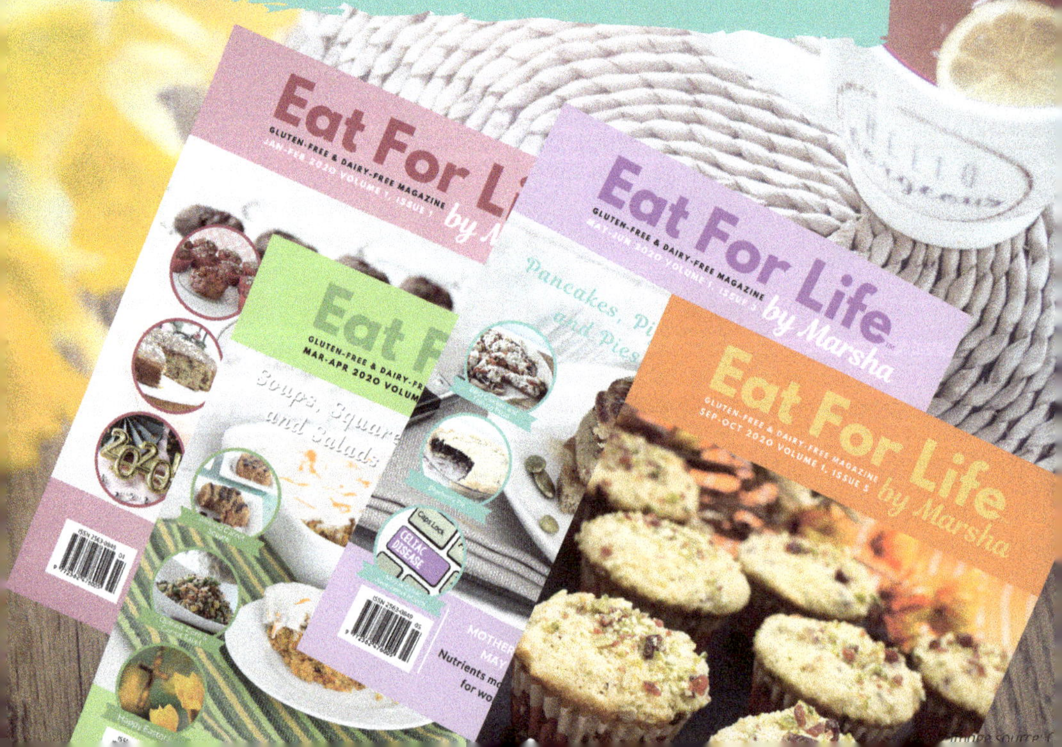

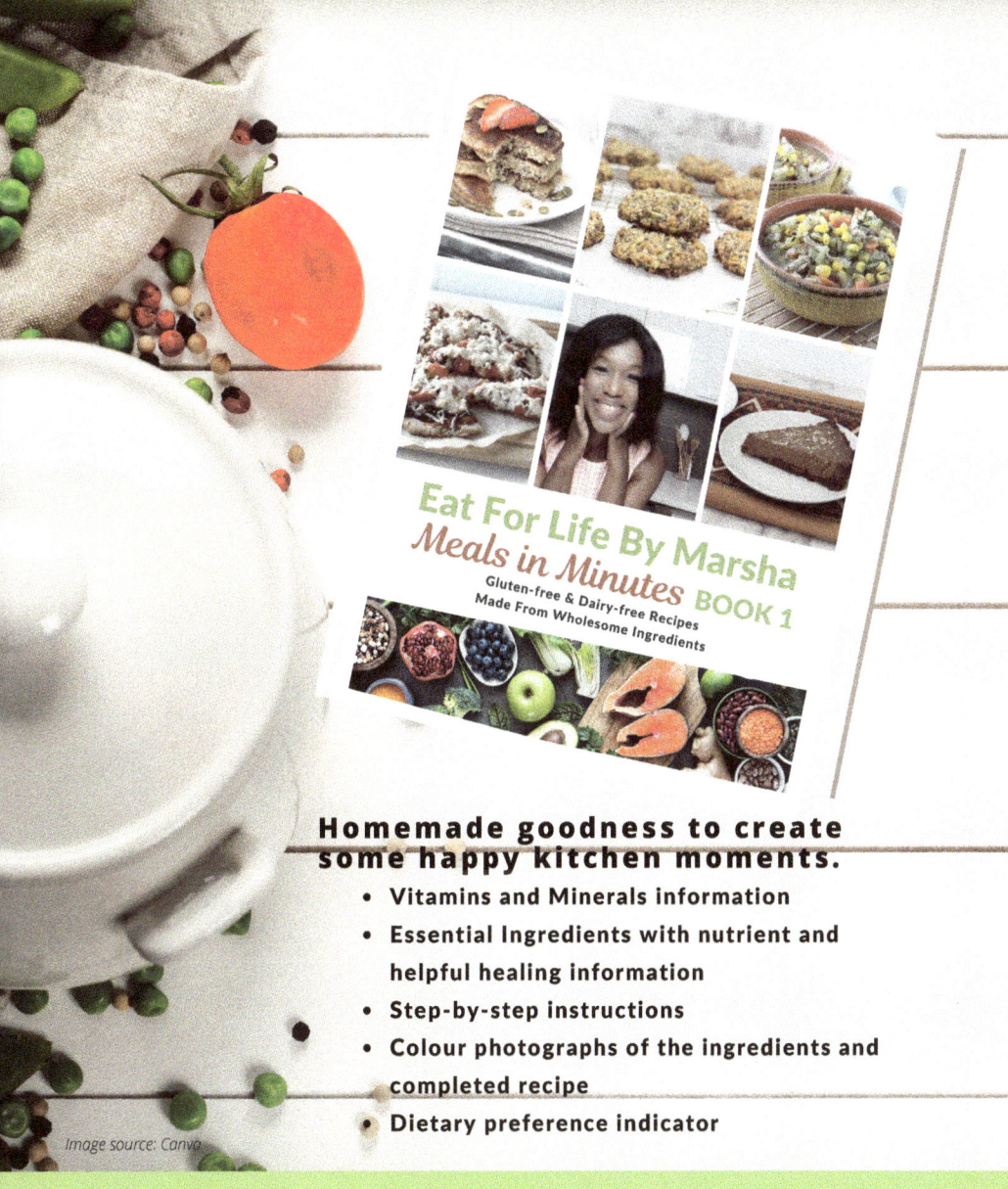

COOKING EQUIVALENT MEASUREMENT

Dry/Weight Measure

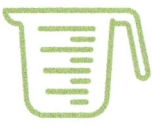

		Ounces	Pounds	Metric
1/16 teaspoon	a dash			
1/8 teaspoon or less	a pinch or 6 drops			.5 ml
1/4 teaspoon	15 drops			1 ml
1/2 teaspoon	30 drops			2 ml
1 teaspoon	1/3 tablespoon	1/6 ounce		5 ml
3 teaspoons	1 tablespoon	1/2 ounce		14 grams
1 tablespoon	3 teaspoons	1/2 ounce		14 grams
2 tablespoons	1/8 cup	1 ounce		28 grams
4 tablespoons	1/4 cup	2 ounces		56.7 grams
5 tablespoons pus 1 teaspoon	1/3 cup	2.6 ounces		75.6 grams
8 tablespoons	1/2 cup	4 ounces	1/4 pound	113 grams
10 tablespoons plus 2 teaspoons	2/3 cup	5.2 ounces		151 grams
12 tablespoons	3/4 cup	6 ounces	.375 pound	170 grams
16 tablespoons	1 cup	8 ounces	.500 or 1/2 pound	225 grams

Liquid or Volume Measurements

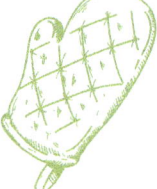

Jigger or measure	1 1/2 or 1.5 fluid ounces		3 tablespoons	45 ml
1 cup	8 fluid ounces	1/2 pint	16 tablespoons	237 ml
2 cups	16 fluid ounces	1 pint	32 tablespoons	474 ml
4 cups	32 fluid ounces	1 quart	64 tablespoons	946 .4
2 pints	32 fluid ounces	1 quart	4 cups	946
4 quarts	128 fluid ounces	1 gallon	16 cups	3.785 liters

Oven Temperatures

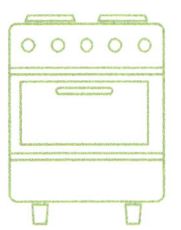

Fahrenheit (Degrees)	Celsius	Gas Mark (Imperial)	Description
225	105	1/3	very cool
250	120	1/2	
275	130	1	cool
300	150	2	
325	165	3	very moderate
350	180	4	moderate
375	190	5	
400	200	6	moderately hot
425	220	7	hot
450	230	8	
475	245	9	very hot

www.ingramcontent.com/pod-product-compliance
Lightning Source LLC
Chambersburg PA
CBHW051552010526
44118CB00022B/2681